Heal Your

Body, Mind, and Spirit

Reviews

This book is going to change the nutrition industry! I've never read a book about nutrition that so thoughtfully connects the dots on how food fits into our overall health picture like this book does. Renata has a fresh, unique perspective that is missing from the health industry and this book provides a beautiful model for anyone searching for answers to discover missing pieces to their health, want to learn a different approach to nutrition, or are curious about learning about their body on a deeper, more holistic level.

Dr. Samantha Chernak, DPT
Holistic Physical Therapist
and Women's Strength Coach

This book is what has been missing from the conversation on health and healing. Renata's way of explaining spirituality makes it easy to understand and relatable. I've tried many of the recipes and they were all delicious, simple ingredients and so nourishing. Renata so eloquently describes how to use food to balance your chakras and the recipes reflect it. These are just a few of the many tools and techniques Renata shares throughout this book. This book will change how you are thinking about your health and wellness in the best, most magical way possible.

Mary Hopper
Author, OT, Business Coach

Heal Your
Body, Mind, and Spirit

Your Ultimate Guide
to nourishing your body,
transforming your mindset,
and developing a stronger
spiritual connection

Renata Trebing
INTUITIVE NUTRITION COACH

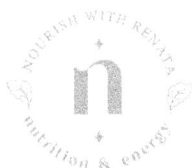

n

NOURISH WITH RENATA

nutrition & energy

PUBLICATIONS

*Heal Your Body, Mind, and Spirit: Your Ultimate Guide
to nourishing your body, transforming your mindset,
and developing a stronger spiritual connection*
By Renata Trebing

Published by Nourish with Renata Publications
Texas, USA

www.nourishwithrenata.com

Contact publisher for bulk orders and permission requests.

Cover design & formatting and interior book design
by Leesa Ellis of 3 ferns books ↦ www.3fernsbooks.com

Interior book formatting by Erin Marie Stirk

Illustrations by Ayesha Santos

Printed in the United States of America.

ISBN (Paperback): 979-8-218-07329-9
ISBN (Hardback): 979-8-218-10253-1

Table of Contents

Foreword

There is an awakening happening.

More and more people are becoming aware that getting healthy is not just about growing muscles and having no body fat.

Our bodies go through so much turmoil and stress each day—from the foods we eat to our jobs, our relationships, and our environment. The amount of stress, toxins, and inflammation seems to grow every single day.

What many people haven't fully recognized is that all of these things have a huge impact on our day-to-day health. This impact can compound if we do not take steps to acknowledge, mitigate, and even prevent them from leaving deep scars in our wellbeing again.

It is time that we start recognizing that our health is not just physical—it is mental, emotional, and spiritual too.

To be healthy is to heal all facets of us as beings: our physical, mental, emotional, and spiritual selves.

In this book, my intention is to help you understand how your physical and energetic self can be used to your greatest advantage to help you heal so that you can become healthier in all areas of life.

This is a truly intuitive journey. It is about getting more and more in tune with who you are. It is about bringing together the science and the spiritual so that you can elevate into the healthiest and happiest you—inside and out.

It is time to heal your body, mind and spirit.

Let food be
thy medicine
and let medicine
be thy food.

– HIPPOCRATES,
FATHER OF MODERN MEDICINE

Introduction

I couldn't even sit down. The pain was so much that it was making it hard to sit at my desk to work. Of course, my co-worker was in the same office as me, but I couldn't let her know that I was in so much pain—let alone tell her that the pain was in my right butt cheek!

As soon as my husband Cody came home, I was desperate to get him to help me. I couldn't understand why I was feeling so much pain. At first, I thought the pain was from a glute workout I had done the previous day, but after stretching and foam rolling, the pain just got worse. Then I noticed a little rash that looked like it had bruises all around it. I couldn't remember if I had fallen down or if I had bumped into something. All I knew was that the pain was almost too much to bear.

Cody looked at the rash and instantly said, "You need to talk to a doctor."

In the next thirty minutes, I was on the phone with my doctor. We had taken a couple of photos of the rash and as soon as my doctor saw it, he said three words that I honestly never thought I would hear.

"You have shingles."

I was completely floored. I had never in a million years thought I would get shingles. Wasn't that something old people got? How did this happen?

My doctor agreed this was unusual. "I would have never expected someone with your health at your age to get shingles. You need to look into this after you finish a course of antiviral medication."

I quickly got started on a ten-day course of these medications. I do think that it helped to clear up my shingles relatively quickly, and it probably helped stop the spreading of shingles too. But it absolutely tore up my stomach. If I took the medication on an empty stomach, or even if I ate a light meal, I would be running to the bathroom with horrible stomach pains and diarrhea. Towards the end of the course of medication, I had to take a trip out of town and at times it was miserable having to feel so much pain but have to act like everything was okay.

Ultimately, the shingles was a wake-up call. It was the moment where I realized that even though I might appear to be healthy on the outside, something inside of me was not right and my body was screaming out to be heard.

I had to figure out what was wrong with me.

This book is a culmination of all the research and experimentation that I did on myself to intuitively heal my body, mind, and spirit. During the months I spent working on myself, I found out some hard truths that I had been ignoring, but also realized some powerful actions that I, and you, can take to bring peace and balance to our physical, mental, emotional, and spiritual health.

If the COVID pandemic has taught us anything, it is that our health is the greatest investment that we can make. And it is an account that we can deposit into every single day. I hope that this book will help you to start making those deposits into the most important bank in the world—You.

Are you ready to begin your healing journey? Let's start today!

Thank you!

Renata

The 5 Levels of Healing

When I heard about the five levels of healing, I have to say that I was skeptical. I mean, isn't healing just for the physical body? Isn't that why we go to doctors and take medicine?

But as I learned more about the five levels of healing, I started to understand it better because it correlated with the experiences that I had in my life when it came to not only healing my physical body, but my mental, emotional, and spiritual wellbeing too.

Several years ago, I stumbled across personal development, through the one and only Mel Robbins. I had seen her TEDx speech[1] on Youtube and something clicked in me. It really made sense to me the things that she was saying about the 5 Second Rule. I started going down the rabbit hole of personal development, and realized that there was a whole other world that I hadn't discovered. I was, of course, familiar with people who were improving their lives through getting fit and eating more wholesome foods, but I realized that there was a layer of improving your life beneath the physical layer. This was when I realized the power of the mind, how this has a huge effect on my personal development, and how I could train myself to look at situations with a totally new perspective. I was finally able to see my own mental strength and how this, along with the physical transformation or through making different choices with food and exercise, could actually work together to start healing the body and mind at the same time.

Sometime later, I started to hear people talking about meditation. It took me a long while to try meditation, because, once again, I was skeptical. And even after I tried it, it took me a long time to understand the benefits of meditation. I realized that I wasn't seeing the benefits of meditation until I was meditating for a longer period of time each day. I started to experience a sense of calm and peace during meditation—a stillness of my mind that was welcomed. It helped me to experience a pause before acting, or reacting, in any situation that happened during the day. Of course, I wasn't perfect every time, but I noticed within myself a certain shift was happening. I was becoming more and more aware.

More recently, I'd discovered breathwork and kundalini yoga. Both of these techniques helped me open up my mind more to the idea of the energetic body. If you've never heard of the energetic body before, and you're starting to really question why you picked up this book, don't worry because I was really skeptical of this idea too. However, even though my brain was questioning this idea, my experience told me something different. During breathwork and kundalini yoga, I was able to feel the sensation of energy running through my body—feel the increase or expansion of energy—by practicing these techniques. Both techniques helped me to cope with the stresses of life and gave me solace or comfort when my physical reality couldn't. Breathwork and kundalini yoga have also had a huge impact on my spiritual connection since it is common for both techniques to help you see or experience a profound realization during the practice. It may even ignite your imagination and see visual images behind your eyelids that you may not be able to explain.

All of my experiences over the past several years had essentially taught me the five levels of healing without me even realizing it. But I needed to experience these things so that I could see the evidence of these layers of healing in my life. And that is why I want to share these levels with you today.

Dr. Dietrich Klinghardt[2], a German holistic doctor, founded the five levels of healing as a systematic model to help us understand the various layers of healing. This knowledge can be helpful when, for instance, physical symptoms appear but physical treatment doesn't seem to help. In these cases, there is often a separate healing level that is needed in order for the physical symptoms to be healed. I have seen this be the case with many people who have autoimmune conditions that are not effectively treated or healed with medication. Instead, functional medicine doctors, or functional nutritionists, are all about helping the patient heal with food, supplements, medicines as well as holistic health practices that I will discuss later in this book. This combination of methods is proving to be more and more effective because it considers the person's whole range of health, not just the physical body. Our bodies, minds, and spirits are all uniquely connected, so it is impossible to treat just the body and consider that all aspects of the human are being healed. It is so much more important, and so needed, to consider the whole person's wellbeing in order to attain true healing—inside and out.

What are the 5 Levels of Healing?

The first level: the Physical Body

This is the level that we are most familiar with. Treating this level includes things like lab testing, medication, and physical manipulation like chiropractic or osteopathic work. Dr. Klinghardt also created Autonomic Response Testing, ART, which is a variety of testing—such as mineral and heavy metal testing, genetic testing, gut and microbiome testing etc—that can help determine what in the physical body may be experiencing disease.

The second level: the Energy Body

This level includes the nervous system, which plays a role in all aspects of our health and wellbeing. The nervous system guides us in automatic functions like breathing as well as complex processes like feelings, emotions, memory, reading, thinking, etc. As we know, all cells in our body utilize energy to function. The energetic body exists within the physical body and is often described with terms like energy centers (chakras) or meridians (energy lines that run through the body). More to come on both of those terms later in this book. Therapies that can help the energy body are acupuncture, meditation, kundalini yoga, and qi gong, which is a Chinese medicine technique that uses slow movement of the body and breath to regulate the body and mind.

The third level: the Mental Body

This level includes the conscious and subconscious mind. Our thoughts create our reality, and yet many people do not acknowledge the power that their minds have that affect our perception and reality. Therapies that can assist this level are homeopathy, mental field therapy, ART, and applied psycho-neurobiology. I also believe that meditation, visualization, and cognitive behavioral therapy can be helpful here.

The fourth level: the Intuitive Body

When I heard about this level, I knew I was on the right track! I had subconsciously known that the intuitive body was something that needed to be understood in order to heal or elevate to the next level of wellness. This level includes intuition, subconscious programming, dreams, and symbology. People have varying levels of awareness of this level of the body. Some people are starting to recognize how their intuition can help them in making decisions, and we will build upon this idea in the Nourish Your Spirit section. Therapies that can help develop awareness of this level are psychotherapy, numerology, astrology, applied psycho-neurobiology, and color and sound therapy.

The fifth level: the Spiritual Body

This is the level of healing that we must all approach on our own, in our own way. It is a deeply personal experience. Spirituality can mean different things to different people. The way in which we connect with who you may call God, The Universe, Source, or a high-er power—if you believe in that—is your own journey to take. Many people find prayer, journaling, and deep meditation to be particu-larly helpful in cultivating a spiritual practice.

I hope that after reading about the five levels of healing, there is a part of you that resonates with this based on your own experiences. The Physical Body, level 1, is the outermost level that is most often treated and more easily understood by most people. But as you dive deeper into a diagnosis or into wanting to truly understand and heal yourself, you may recognize that there is so much more to you than just your physical body. The ultimate healing occurs when we acknowledge the healing that is needed from the innermost level, your Spiritual Body, first, all the way to your outermost level, your Physical Body.

Explained another way, physical symptoms are actually the last indication that there is something that needs to be healed on the other levels. In fact, this was why I believe that I had shingles. I was ignoring the other signs that there was healing needed on levels two through five. My body had to have a massive outbreak in order to get me to pay attention and do some major healing from the outside all the way into the Spiritual Body.

The takeaway from learning about the five levels of healing is don't wait for your symptoms to show up on your physical body. If you believe that something is not aligned with any of your other levels, then pay attention and take the steps to heal them. If you don't, you may end up like me, with your body screaming out for attention, so that you can finally begin your healing journey on all five levels.

▰▰▰▶ Action Items

Knowledge can be powerful if you take action. In each of the following sections, I encourage you to read and implement the following action items to get the most transformation from the guidance in this book.

Write down your responses to the following questions. It may be helpful to have a dedicated journal for the work that you will do throughout this book and the insights that you have.

* What resonated with you regarding the five levels of healing? How does this relate with your own healing journey thus far? On the physical level? Or any other levels?

* What symptoms are you currently experiencing? What level of healing do you believe these symptoms stem from?

* What is your health and wellness goal?

Beginning Your Journey

I have divided this book into three parts:

Part 1: Heal Your Body
Part 2: Heal Your Mind
Part 3: Heal Your Spirit

Each of these parts are integral to healing the whole person. One part cannot exist to its greatest elevation without the other parts. I believe that health and wellness is when all three parts of a person can be healed and elevated to their next level of awareness and wellbeing.

In Part One, Heal Your Body, I will focus on nutrition and tangible physical aspects that I went through to heal my gut, immune system, etc. This section of the book deals primarily with level one healing of the Physical Body, as explained in the five levels of healing.

In Part Two, we will focus on mindset and how to heal the thoughts that may be keeping you from reaching your health goals. I'll also discuss the gut-brain axis and how nutrition can impact your brain health. This section covers level three of the five levels of healing.

And finally in Part Three, I will discuss the energetic body, chakras, and healing your energy centers as well as sharing my favorite holistic health practices to help align your body. This section covers levels two, four and five.

In each part, I will also be sharing tools to help you connect with and improve your intuition. As Carolyn Holden says, our intuition is our greatest healing tool. Sometimes we just need a little guidance to help us unlock that potential within us. I believe that our intuition is always guiding us. We just need to learn how to listen.

I recommend reading this book in order since it is sometimes easier to start with the tangible, physical things first before delving into the mind and spirit work. But please know that whatever part of the book you feel drawn to, that is what you may need in that moment. Follow your intuition and what it is telling you.

Let's begin healing your body, mind, and spirit!

PART 1

Heal Your Body

Shingles was no joke. The rash was both itchy and painful. It often felt like sharp pinpricks. Anytime I started to feel my stress levels rising, it created a cascade of electrified pinpricks coursing through my body, even in places where the rash wasn't physically present.

Not only that, the antiviral medications really affected my stomach. If I didn't take the medicine with food, I would have horrible stomach upset and diarrhea. That is the last thing you want to be dealing with when you also have pain radiating from the rash!

It was apparent that my physical body needed to heal from both the shingles and the antiviral medication.

∽ ∝

Healing your body is where we most often start. You might have a cold, stomach upset, or just want your body to look a different way. Healing your body might sound like an arduous task, but honestly it is about one principle: being mindful about how you treat your physical body.

Everything that you put into your body is affecting your cells. Through scientific research[3], we know that every single piece of food, drink, or the chemicals that enter your body have the opportunity to influence how your DNA is expressed. This is called epigenetics.

Epigenetic mechanisms begin in utero, when the fetus is developing in the uterus. Any exposure to harmful environmental toxins can potentially hinder the epigenome from developing properly, which may lead the individual to develop a disease later in life.

The converse is also true. The foods that we put into our bodies now can potentially protect our bodies from developing disease. Understanding the impact of foods that we absorb can then become useful methods of preventing disease and improving overall wellbeing.

Medication can have a huge impact on our bodies. There are many medications that have a long-lasting positive impact for people, and other well-intentioned meds may have a myriad of side effects. This was exactly what I had experienced. I saw benefits from taking the medication to stop the shingles rash from spreading, but the downside was the incessant and sometimes painful stomach upset issues.

So, after I finished my course of medication to treat shingles, it was obvious that my gut needed some serious healing. I called this my Intuitive Gut Healing Journey. I do believe that most people have gut issues, but they haven't taken the time to think about what their gut issues are or what to do about it.

If you are curious if your gut may need some extra healing too, here are some common signs of a gut health issue.

* Irregular or painful bowel movements

* Very loose bowel movements e.g. diarrhea

* Pain or discomfort when trying to use the restroom

* Frequent bloating

* Frequent gas

* Difficulty passing stool

✳ Pain or discomfort after eating certain foods: I go into a little more detail around determining your intolerances in my previous book, *Nourish Your Body: A 30-Day Healthy and Delicious Meal Plan,* and accompanying journal, *Track Your Food, Change Your Life.*

If you are experiencing one or more of the symptoms listed, or have concerns that there is something wrong with your gut, today is the perfect time to start taking steps to heal your gut.

Healing the gut can seem like such a big mission, but honestly, it just starts with a simple step forward each day and then building upon that habit whenever you feel capable. You can continue with this habit and add another habit to it.

The Importance of Gut Health

Gut health is a popular buzzword and for good reason. But why is gut health so important? Here are a few reasons why gut health needs to be at the top of your health list for daily improvement:

✳ **Immunity:** The gut has a huge impact on how effective our immune systems are. In fact, over 70% of our immune system is located in the gut itself.

✳ **Gut-brain axis:** This is a special connection between the gut and the brain where the health of the gut can feed the health of the brain, and vice versa.

✳ **Digestive health:** The most obvious reason why we improve our gut health is because we want to ensure we are having good digestive health. Most people think this means that we have regular bowel movements, which is true. But good digestive health also means reduced bloating, eliminating pain in the digestive system, eliminating toxins from the body more effectively etc.

There are two main steps to improving gut health. The first step is to find out your gut health triggers—the foods that irritate your gut and cause upset stomach, poor digestive motility or constipation, excessive gas and bloating, stomach pain either during or before bowel movements, etc.

Some of the most common foods that irritate the gut health of many people are:

1. **Refined sugars:** We have all heard the negative impact that sugars can have on our health. Sugar can cause fermentation in the belly, which then causes inflammation. Excessive and prolonged inflammation can then lead to other chronic illnesses like diabetes, obesity etc. However, sugar is often in many things that we eat, especially refined and packaged foods. That is why, during my intuitive healing journey, I opted to remove sugars, alcohol, and sweeteners from my eating plan to observe the effect that this had on my gut. I realized that I was reliant on sweeteners to make things taste, well, sweet! This is a totally natural human desire since we have been bred to like sweet foods. This doesn't mean that you can never eat sweet foods again. But for the purposes of healing your gut, you may want to take a short break from refined sugars or artificial sweeteners to see what impact that has on your gut health.

2. **Alcohol:** Alcohol is another thing that causes a lot of gut distress. Some studies[5] have shown that alcohol can negatively affect the balance of good and bad bacteria in the gut. For me, I also didn't really like the taste of alcohol, nor did I like the way it made me feel, so I had no problem not drinking alcohol. However, I know for many people it is something they enjoy doing or they

have grown up using alcohol as a relaxation or social-bonding method. If you are ready to heal your body, you may consider reducing or removing alcohol for a certain timeframe, say thirty days, and see how you feel. You can then slowly reintroduce it after that time has passed. If you feel some resistance to avoiding alcohol for this timeframe, it may be helpful to ask yourself:

a. Why do you drink alcohol?

b. Where did this habit come from?

c. How did you learn about drinking alcohol?

d. What was your first experience of drinking alcohol?

e. How does it make you feel and why are these feelings important/not important to you?

f.   How do you know when you've had enough alcohol? Do you stop at this point or not?

g. When do you feel drawn to drinking alcohol?

These questions may be helpful so that you get to the underlying reason why you may be feeling this resistance. You can also apply the same questions to any of the other common gut irritants listed in this section.

1. **Artificial sweeteners:** There are a lot of artificial sweeteners on the market now that are questionable regarding how they will impact your body when used consistently and for the long term. This is the risk with artificial sweeteners, especially those created from synthetic ingredients as opposed to ones derived from plant foods. Unfortunately, at this time, we just don't know for sure what is going to happen later on in life if we continue to consume artificial sweeteners, especially in large quantities. In time, I do believe there will be more scientific studies on the long-term impact

of artificial sweeteners. However, during my intuitive gut healing journey, I opted to remove artificial sweeteners as a way of reducing inflammation.

The second step to improving gut health is to add more of the foods to your eating plan that help foster the growth of the "good" gut bacteria or probiotics, as well as integrating other holistic health practices that reduce stress and reinforce gut health improvements.

How to Heal Your Gut

Here are the seven daily ways that I intuitively healed my gut during my intuitive gut healing journey:

Step 1: Hydration

This is always the first step! Hydration is usually the easiest habit to start since you typically can do it without having to purchase any other ingredients.

Water is vital for all of our organs to function properly. We now know that even a one percent reduction in hydration can cause our mental cognition to be affected. This means that even if you are slightly dehydrated, you may find that your thoughts are a little foggy or it's harder to remember things.

Hydration also impacts our gut health. When we are adequately hydrated, it impacts the mucosal lining of the gut and the balance of good bacteria. Hydration also makes it easier for waste to move through the digestive system.

How much water should you drink? I always tell my clients to aim to drink at least half of their body weight in ounces of water each day. For example, if you weigh 200lbs, then you would aim to drink about 100oz of water each day. This can be affected by any medications that may be a diuretic (caffeinated beverages like coffee or tea are diuretics) or if you sweat a lot, either through exercise or your work so you may want to increase your hydration levels.

If you've calculated the amount of water recommended for you to drink daily, and you have realized that what you're currently drinking is way lower than your goal, don't worry! Here are a few tips to help you build up to your goal water intake:

* **Step up your water intake gradually** by drinking one extra bottle/glass of water each day as soon as you get up in the morning. The sooner you get this new habit done in your day, the less procrastination you'll experience and the more accomplishment you'll feel.

* **Use a straw to drink your water:** Drinking from a straw creates a vacuum to draw water into the straw then into your mouth. This makes drinking water much more efficient because you're not taking in as much air while you're drinking. Just think about when you're drinking from a glass. Air is flowing into your mouth at the same time as the drink. To avoid this, and to increase the amount of water you're drinking daily, try a straw. There are many great reusable straws that fit most lids too.

* **Flavor your water:** If you're bored with the water you're drinking, try to add a little flavor. The easiest way to do this is to add things like a few slices of lemons, oranges or limes into your water and let it infuse for several minutes. Other variations include sliced ginger, basil, lemon, berries, cucumber, mint, and cinnamon. Have fun testing out the different flavor combos.

* **Find the water temperature that works best for you:** Different people have said to me they cannot drink ice cold

water, or conversely, there are other people who say ice cold water is the only water they can drink. I encourage you to figure out or test what temperature of water you prefer. It is important to figure this out so that you know exactly what water you can drink a lot of at the end of the day, just in case you didn't hit your water goal yet.

An obvious occurrence when you start drinking a lot of water is that you will have to go to the restroom a lot. This is just a part of it. But it will help you determine if you are drinking enough water. If your urine is a dark yellow color, this is an indication that you are not drinking enough water and are potentially dehydrated.

If your urine is very light yellow or close to clear, this indicates that you are likely drinking enough water for your body and to replenish your electrolyte stores.

The great thing is that your body will actually get used to the new amount of water you are drinking. So, I recommend sticking with your new water goal intake number or continuing to step up your water intake over time. Your body will soon become accustomed to it.

If you find that you are drinking a lot of water but still feeling parched, this can be an indication that your electrolyte balance is off. You can aid this by adding a pinch of pink Himalayan salt to your water or getting an electrolyte supplement (preferably one with no sugar) to help rebalance your electrolytes. Alternatively, just make sure to salt your foods adequately.

■■➤ **Action Items**

Answer the following questions in your journal:

* How much water am I currently drinking each day on average?

* How much water should I be drinking each day?

* If needed, what one action can I take today to increase my water intake?

Step 2: Eat more fiber

Fiber is important for your body, and not just to make sure you have regular bowel movements. Fiber is also the food for the good bacteria in your gut. We get fiber from all plant foods, like fruits, vegetables, nuts and seeds. One of the first things that I did when healing my gut was to increase my fiber intake. Experts recommend that women aim for at least 25g of fiber daily, while men should consume around 35g of fiber per day minimum.

Prior to getting shingles, I had been tracking my food intake using an app, and felt confident that my fiber numbers were reaching 25g daily. However, I knew that I could improve my fiber numbers up to 40g per day while also aiming for lots of variety. Having variety in your fiber sources helps to feed a larger variety of the good gut bacteria. I like to have about thirty different plant foods each week. This is actually easy to do especially when you choose a couple of new plant foods from the grocery store to try every week.

Fiber helps us feel fuller for longer. Studies[6] have shown that people who eat more fiber, typically have a lower risk of obesity, heart disease, and diabetes. Not to mention, more fiber for the good gut bacteria to grow and thrive. Improving your gut health will also help to improve immunity, cognitive function, aid in achieving a healthy weight, and help you live longer too.

Lastly, more fiber means more regular bowel movements, assuming that you are also drinking plenty of water with it too. If you are still having issues with digestion, it may be time to seek professional guidance.

➡ Action Items

* How much fiber are you eating now? You may consider using a food tracking app to determine this, such as MyFitnessPal. Another way to determine this is to see how many plant foods you eat during a typical week.

* What can you do today to help you to increase your fiber intake? Eg: adding an extra handful of vegetables to your plate, making a fiber-rich smoothie (see a recipe on page 133), including a fiber supplement in your eating plan etc.

Step 3: Probiotics

The gut contains what are often termed as "good" and "bad" bacteria. Probiotics is the scientific term for the good bacteria. We want to make sure we have lots of good bacteria in our gut to help with more effective digestion, improve immunity, improve the connection between the gut and the brain, and so much more.

Getting a daily source of probiotics ensures that we are getting more good bacteria into our bodies. The good bacteria help to eliminate the bad bacteria, restoring the balance to your gut microbiome.

You can get probiotics from a number of sources. Firstly, you can get probiotics in fermented foods, such as kimchi and sauerkraut, as well as kefir, kombucha, yogurt, etc, or you can invest in a daily probiotic capsule or a powder.

A probiotic supplement is simply a strain or multiple strains of healthy gut bacteria that can be used to aid your existing gut microbiome. The most common bacteria used in supplements are Lactobacillus and Bifidobacterium. Probiotics may also contain the yeast Saccharomyces boulardii.

Nowadays, there are so many options for probiotics, such as probiotics for women over fifty or a daily probiotic powder for kids. Generally speaking, finding a probiotic supplement can be a little bit of trial and error, especially if you don't get special gut bacteria lab tests. Please note that the higher the dosage, or Colony Forming Units (CFUs), of the probiotics you take, the more powerful the probiotics may be. Some probiotics need to be kept in the fridge since they are active or live cultures.

Probiotics are generally considered safe for most people and can be a great addition to your current supplementation regimen. However, if you have a medical condition, it is recommended to speak to your medical professional before starting a course of probiotics.

➡ Action Items

* Do you currently take a probiotic supplement or incorporate probiotic-rich foods in your eating plan?

* If not, what is one thing you can do today to increase your probiotic intake?

Step 4: Get more sleep

This was a big one for me!

I knew that I was not getting enough sleep each night—at the time, I was sleeping around five hours per night—but I didn't feel like I needed any more sleep than that! Until I got the shingles. I knew that the stress that I was carrying wasn't getting released through sleep because my sleep schedule was so short. So, I immediately made sure to start getting at least seven hours of sleep per night.

Not only did this help to reduce my cortisol levels (the stress hormone) but it also allowed my gut time to digest any remaining food, regulate blood sugar levels, and produce more serotonin, the feel-good hormone. More sleep also meant a heightened immune system. So, sleep is truly a powerful tool to help to heal the body. More on that in Part Two: Heal Your Mind.

▰▰▶ Action Items

* How much sleep do you typically get each night?

* Are you getting quality sleep? Or are you woken up many times in the night?

* How much sleep would you like to get?

Step 5: Daily Self-care Practices

Self-care is anything that you can do to help take care of your physical, mental, emotional, and spiritual health. I like to call this "filling up your proverbial cup." Self-care can help you in so many ways, e.g. increases your resilience, improves your ability to manage stress, living longer, as well as having more peace, joy, and happiness.

I honestly thought that my self-care practice was pretty good before I got shingles, but shingles showed me that I really didn't. I was holding onto so much stress from other people, work, my personal life, etc that I didn't even realize the amount of stress that I was under (more on this in Part two). So, in addition to sleep, I committed to finding ways to destress as much as possible through self-care. Some nights that meant putting the computer away and watching a TV show; other nights it was reading a book, and sometimes it was just going to sleep early. Whatever your self-care practice is, make sure that you commit to doing so regularly or, ideally, every day. It really shocked me that I didn't know how much stress I was under until I started my daily self-care practices.

■■■➤ **Action Items**

* Do you have any daily self-care practices? What are they?

* Do you feel like these practices are truly enough to reduce your stress and fill up your proverbial cup?

Step 6: Know Your Food Intolerances

Most people don't realize the effect certain foods have on their bodies. I, for one, didn't realize my own food intolerance until it was forced upon me. When my first child, Olivia, was born, I was breast-feeding her and didn't understand what was causing her digestion problems. Our pediatrician suggested that perhaps Olivia was allergic or intolerant to something I was eating, and it was being passed to her through the breast milk. Little did I know that the most common allergen for infants is actually dairy. So, I removed dairy from my diet and was amazed at the difference that I saw in Olivia! Her digestive issues improved and then disappeared. She was also able to sleep better through the night. That made me, the sleep-deprived new mom, so happy! But, also, I realized that my bloating and digestive discomfort were going away too. It was then that I finally understood that dairy did not agree with my body.

Have you ever felt that there was a food that didn't agree with your body? This can be a great indicator for a food intolerance or mild allergy. The easiest way of determining your own food intolerances is to simply keep a journal or note of what you eat during the day and how you feel afterwards. You can also use my journal, *Track Your Food, Change Your Life,* available on Amazon, to do this. Do this for a few weeks in order to observe a trend with any foods that are causing feelings of discomfort, bloating, stomach upset, skin rashes, etc. This can give you a good indication of the foods that your body is not tolerating well.

Some of the most common food intolerances are wheat, gluten, soy, and dairy. Some people also have intolerances to certain nuts, seeds, fruits, and vegetables. Since some of these foods are considered generally healthy, that is why it is so important to figure out the foods that your body agrees with or disagrees with. Once you know these foods, you can aim to reduce or eliminate them from your eating plan completely. Do this for a few weeks or even up to a month and notice how differently you feel. If you do try an elimination diet, I highly recommend doing this under the supervision of a professional in order to keep a good eye on any potential reactions or changes in mood and energy that you may experience.

I recently had a client who went through a thirty-day elimination diet program where she removed allergens from her diet. Within the first five days, she had already lost four pounds of water retention from bloating and inflammation. She felt so much lighter and, with the increased fiber in her diet, her digestive system was finally working well so that she was feeling better each day. By the end of the thirty days, she was down over six pounds and lost two and a half inches around her whole body. She also commented that there were areas on her body where the swelling had reduced so much that she could actually see the scars that were the original culprit for the damage. Previously, the inflammation in her body was so bad that the original scars could not be seen.

Not only that, this client started to experience massive physical healing. Her bowel movements were not difficult or painful, the inflammation in her body had reduced significantly so even her Thai massage therapist recognized how much easier it was to work on her body, her PMS symptoms reduced or disappeared completely. She even commented that she was having greater mental clarity and found enjoyment in the kitchen again. I do believe that these improvements happened because she worked to heal her gut through removing the allergens that were causing irritation to her gut lining.

As a result, her mindset changed towards food and cooking, and her cognitive improvements were palpable too.

▰▰▰▶ Action Items

✻ What are your food allergies or intolerances?

✻ Are there any foods that you feel do not agree with you?

✻ If you do not know which foods may be triggering a negative reaction with you, I highly recommend starting a simple food journal to write down what you ate and how it made you feel during and/or afterwards. Continue doing this for three to four weeks then look back at your journal to find any trends.

The Fab Four

The next step in healing your body is knowing what foods help you feel satiated, energized, and give you all the nutrients that you need.

That is why I love the Fab Four method. The Fab Four is a term coined by Kelly LeVeque, a celebrity nutritionist, and I have seen this method work amazingly on clients to help them lose weight, actually feel full when they eat, and have more sustained energy throughout the day.

You can refer to Kelly's books for a more detailed explanation of the Fab Four, but here is my simplified breakdown.

The Fab Four are four main ingredients you should ideally have on your plate at every meal. When you have these four ingredients, you will feel full after eating (no more starving yourself or feeling deprived), your hormones will become more balanced, your energy levels will be more even, and you may even have the additional benefit of losing weight and inches.

Here are the four ingredients:

✳ **Protein:** The building block of all cells in our bodies. Protein is needed by the body for cellular repair, especially if you are working out. When we exercise, such as lifting weights, we are purposefully tearing the muscle fibers so that they can grow back thicker and stronger. But, if we are not eating enough protein, we actually prevent the body from adequately repairing those muscle fibers. This is because the body aims to find any available fuel source even when additional protein is not consumed. In fact, the body eats away at the existing muscle in order to have enough fuel to keep you moving during the day. So, your hard work of going to the gym is literally getting eaten away by your body! Make sure you eat protein at every meal, and even at snack times too. Protein is also the highest satiating ingredient, which means that it helps you feel fuller than any other ingredient. You can get protein from animal and plant sources, everything from beef, seafood, chickpeas, and broccoli contain protein. Every protein source will have a specific amino acid profile so to prevent any potential deficiencies in amino acids, aim to eat a wide variety of different protein sources.

✳ **Healthy Fats:** When most people hear the word fat, they start fearing they are going to get fat too. Instead, healthy fats are needed by your cells for cell-to-cell communication and the healthy functioning of several hormones. Healthy fats, specifically omega-3, are anti-inflammatory fatty acids that we need to consume from food. Omega-3s also help to prevent depression[7]. When we eat healthy fats, they help to slow digestion which, once again, helps us to feel fuller for longer. Healthy fats can be found in avocados, wild caught salmon, nuts/seeds, any nut/seed oils or butters, coconut oil or coconut etc.

* **Fiber:** We've talked about the massive benefits of fiber already but just to reiterate, fiber helps our digestive system health, and it expands in the digestive tract so that we feel fuller. Most people are not eating enough fiber. In fact, most women that come to me for nutritional coaching are only eating about half of their daily recommended fiber intake. So, remember to get a high volume and lots of different plant foods (fiber comes from all plant foods) in your daily eating so that you get a wide range of fiber. A wide variety of fiber helps foster the growth of the various kinds of good bacteria that exist within the body.

* **Greens:** This is what I believe is often the missing secret ingredient from many people's eating on a day-to-day basis. Greens, such as kale, spinach, bok choy, cabbage, etc are not only fiber powerhouses, but nutritional powerhouses too. Greens contain high levels of iron, antioxidants like glutathione, and help to trigger a certain hunger hormone called Glucagon-Like Peptide-1, GLP-1, that tells your brain that you are feeling full. Without this hormone being triggered, you may not feel that feeling of fullness after eating a meal, and instead be more inclined to eat more than your typical serving size.

The Fab Four doesn't list specifically refined carbohydrates. Why? Because it is so easy to eat an inordinately large amount of carbohydrates and not necessarily feel full. Also, refined carbohydrates tend to have little nutritional value since they are typically removed during processing.

This doesn't mean that you can never have a piece of toast or pasta again, but now you can make different choices and perhaps choose a refined carbohydrate product that has more nutritional value or is in alignment with your specific health and wellness goals.

■■■➤ Action Item

Try the Fab Four method during your next meal and note how full you feel afterwards.

How to Build Your Plate: The Simple Plate Method and the Palm-Fist-Fist Method

Now that you know the Fab Four, the next step is to know how to build your plate. There have been many iterations of what constitutes a healthy plate. From the food pyramid to the My Plate method, more and more scientific research is showing the benefit of being more mindful about what is on our plates and in what quantities.

There are two methods I like to teach my clients about when we are discussing serving sizes. The first is the Simple Plate Method.

The Simple Plate Method

The Simple Plate Method focuses on having a good amount of vegetables on your plate, as opposed to the traditional American plate, which focuses on protein being the center of the plate. While protein is important, I find that most people are completely missing out on or eating significantly low amounts of vegetables on a daily basis. Vegetables are essential for nutrients, vitamins, minerals, fiber, and over six servings of fruits and vegetables per day has been linked to a reduced risk of cancer. So, let's get more veggies into us and see the added benefit of healing our bodies from the inside out.

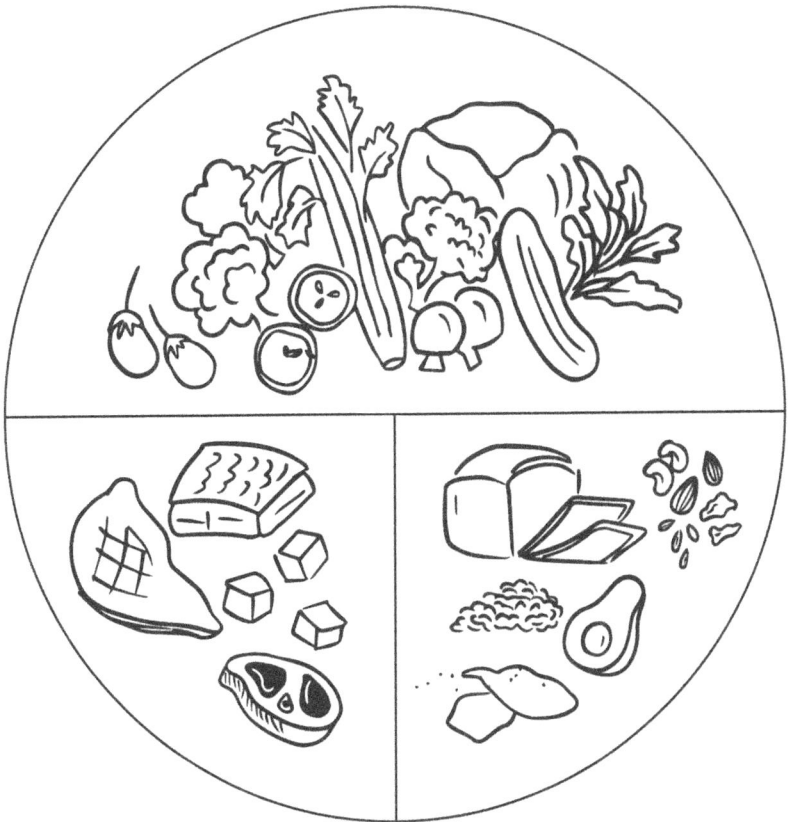

* Your plate can be divided into four equal quadrants.

* For two quadrants, this is where you put your non-starchy vegetables.

* For one quadrant, this is where you place your protein source.

* And for the final quadrant, this is for your healthy fats and any starchy carbohydrates.

This Simple Plate Method has been attributed to improved heart health, reduced cholesterol, and reduced waistlines. It is incredibly easy to use since all you need is a plate. No measuring equipment needed. Of course, there will be times when you have a casserole or a soup and all the ingredients are mixed together. Don't worry! Just use your best estimate on serving sizes and know that one meal doesn't derail you. The next meal is another opportunity to use the Simple Plate method and continue working towards your health and wellness goals.

The Palm-Fist-Fist Method:

This is another easy-to-use method for approximating serving sizes. All you need is one hand. What is great about the Palm-Fist-Fist method is that everyone's hands are generally in proportion to that person's size so this method is easily customizable for each individual.

The Palm-Fist-Fist method is also a great place to start when it comes to determining the portion size of each ingredient that works best for you. For instance, I know that my body prefers a higher amount of protein so I increase my protein serving to two palms as opposed to the generic recommendation for women of one palm of protein. This works for me. You may find that you work better with two fists of non-starchy carbohydrates as opposed to one, or perhaps a two-thumb portion of fat is better for you than one. The Palm-Fist-Fist method provides a baseline of where to start to figure out the food portions that suit your body best.

The Palm-Fist-Fist Method can also be adjusted depending on your particular health goals. For instance, if your goal is weight loss, you might start off with the recommended guidelines and then gradually reduce the starchy carb amount. Or for weight gain, you may increase up to two thumbs of healthy fats right away. The choice is truly yours.

The following is a simple explanation of the Palm-Fist-Fist method.

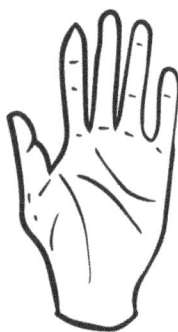

Palm

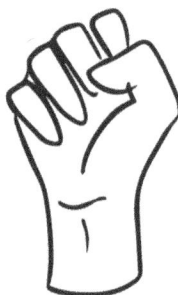

Fist

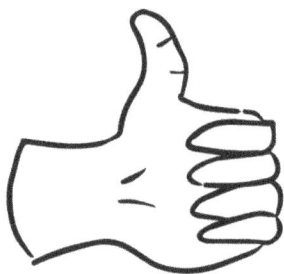

Thumb

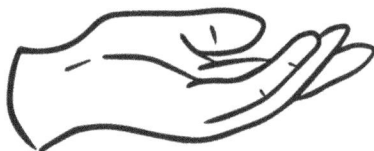

Cupped Hand

✳ **Palm:** This is the approximate amount of protein for your plate. The palm is the area from the heel of your hand to where the fingers and thumb meet the palm. The protein can be roughly the size, shape and thickness of the palm. For women, one palm of protein is recommended whereas for men, two palms of protein is recommended.

✳ **Fist:** The size and shape of your fist is a good approximation for the amount of non-starchy carbohydrates to eat. This includes veggies like broccoli, cauliflower, kale, spinach, watercress, beetroot, radishes, green beans, etc. For women, one fist is recommended, and for men two fists are recommended.

✳ **A cupped hand:** This is the serving for your starchy carbohydrates. These are things like corn, carrots, peas, rice, quinoa, millet etc. For women, one cupped hand is recommended, and for men, two cupped hands are recommended.

✳ **Thumb:** The size and shape of your thumb can help you to approximate a serving of healthy fats. For women, one thumb is recommended, and for men, two thumbs are recommended.

Once again, the Palm-Fist-Fist method is a great way of approximating the serving sizes for food. There will be times when the food is all mixed together like in soups or stews, so just use your best guess for the servings and give yourself grace. Just as I mentioned above, one meal is not going to make or break your progress. Consistent frequent action towards your goals will be more powerful and more effective to get you closer to achieving your health goals.

■■■➤ **Action Items**

Which method above do you think will help you reach your health and wellness goal(s)?

Use that method the next time you make a plate and write down what you notice about the portion sizes, and how you feel after you eat.

Inflammation

One of the most harmful culprits to your body is inflammation. There are two kinds of inflammation:

1. **Acute inflammation:** This is where inflammation occurs at a specific, localized area e.g., when you get a paper cut. The skin around the paper cut gets red, might hurt a little bit, but eventually it heals. No more inflammation.

2. **Chronic inflammation:** This is the inflammation that may occur throughout a larger portion of the body and hangs around, even when we don't recognize it. Chronic inflammation in the body for an extended period of time can often lead to many chronic conditions, such as diabetes, hypertension, obesity, heart conditions etc. Chronic inflammation is often called the silent killer because we tend to accept a low level of discomfort in the body, thinking that it is normal when it really isn't.

As you can see, inflammation can be detrimental to our overall well-being. But where does inflammation come from?

Inflammation can arise from many things, including various foods that we may have a sensitivity or allergy to, stress, lack of sleep, increased environmental toxins—such as cleaning products or from personal care items. Inflammation can even be caused in the body from mold in your house/apartment, animals that you are allergic to, and dust or pollen in the air you breathe.

Reducing inflammation allows your body to lower its immune system response. We can do that by understanding which food groups we have allergies/intolerances to, lowering stress, getting more sleep, and creating a more toxin-free environment too. I'll share more about stress mitigation techniques and sleep later in this book.

You can also help to reduce your inflammation by adding more anti-inflammatory foods, such as wild caught salmon, chia seeds, flax seeds, and omega-3 supplements. Omega-3s are the anti-inflammatory fatty acids that our body does not produce, so we need to make sure that we are consuming Omega-3s regularly to help to lower inflammation in our bodies.

There are three kinds of Omega-3s:

1. Alpha-linolenic acid, ALA
2. Docosahexaenoic acid, DHA
3. Eicosapentaenoic acid, EPA

ALA is found in plant sources such as flaxseeds, walnuts, and chia seeds. The body has to process ALA into DHA and EPA, and the effectiveness and efficiency of this process varies depending on the individual, so you may not be getting the full benefit of the omega-3s if your body is not converting ALA to DHA and EPA.

DHA and EPA are found in animal sources, such as wild-caught fatty fish like salmon, herring, tuna, mackerel, and trout. These two compounds have been found to be the most important and effective compounds for reducing inflammation. EPA supports the heart, immune system, and inflammatory response, while DHA supports the brain, eyes, and the central nervous system.

I often recommend my clients to start incorporating an Omega-3 supplement into their daily routine in addition to increasing their consumption of Omega-3 rich foods into their eating plan. When looking for an Omega-3 supplement, it should contain both EPA and DHA. Omega-3 supplements should be high quality and have minimum toxins, so make sure to research the manufacturer and avoid any fishy-smelling or tasting supplements. If your supplements smell or taste fishy, it is a sign that the fish oils are beginning to degrade and will not be as beneficial for you to consume anymore.

➡ Action Items

* Have you noticed any long-lasting inflammation in your body? Where is it?

* Are you regularly consuming Omega-3 supplements or Omega-3-rich foods?

* If not, what foods or supplements can you start incorporating today/this week?

Final Thoughts on Healing Your Body

Ultimately, healing your body comes down to staying hydrated and fueling and nourishing your body with foods that are wholesome and unrefined. Every morsel of food is impacting your body. This doesn't mean that you can never have chips or cookies again. Instead, I simply suggest being mindful about the food that you put in your body. Ask yourself, why do I feel like eating this? Am I really hungry? Or am I trying to self-soothe my body because of an event that has happened? The key is awareness. And when you have the awareness of the power of food and how it truly has a huge impact on your physical, mental and emotional health, you will begin to look at food in a completely new light as an important element to your healing journey.

━━➤ **Action Items**

Answer the following questions in your journal:

* What are your biggest learnings from this section?

* What can you start implementing today to help heal your body? I suggest adopting one new habit every couple of weeks or every month. This may seem like a slow integration, but when we become thoughtful and purposeful with our habits, we begin to deeply engrain these new habits into our daily way of being. The key is to do this one simple habit consistently. When you feel you have gotten this habit down, start implementing a new habit. This method does take time, and it has been shown to be the most effective at creating sustainable, life-long change to your health and wellbeing.

* Set up a time every week to reflect and see if you have successfully implemented these daily tasks. What can you do to improve your success at this habit? Make it a non-negotiable! Remember, the best investment you can make is in your health.

"Be mindful about what you are thinking and you will create a new reality for yourself."

– RENATA TREBING

PART 2

Heal Your Mind

One of the most important—yet rarely discussed—areas to heal is the mind. Our mind controls our thoughts and beliefs, and in fact, our end results because of it.

We don't often realize it, but our thoughts are influenced by our environment, the books we read, the podcasts we listen to, the news, what our family members say, social media—literally everything! If we are not conscious of the influencing factors, we can start going down negative thought spirals, which can ultimately impact our entire world.

While recovering from shingles, I started to be aware that my thoughts were becoming really negative. I was focusing on the things that really annoyed me, made me upset, frustrated, and overwhelmed. These thoughts kept circling around in my brain for most of the day. I started thinking and feeling like I was a victim of my diagnosis, wondering if I would ever be able to function properly again.

∽ ∾

The Power of the Brain

The brain has two halves, the left side and the right side. Each side of the brain has different functions and processes sensory information in different ways to support these functions.

The left side of the brain is responsible for reasoning, explanations, speech, and beliefs. This side of the brain is analytical and logical.

The right side of the brain is responsible for creativity, consciousness, peace, and calm. This side of the brain is all about visualization, feelings, and other nonverbal cues.

Both sides of the brain can work together and one side of the brain can become dominant in certain situations. The key is understanding how each side of the brain works and when you want to use one side more than the other.

For instance, when trying to understand a new concept, the left side of the brain takes over, looking for evidence to explain and help you understand the new information. The right side of the brain is quieted temporarily so that you can focus on absorbing and understanding this new idea. Alternatively, when in meditation, the right side of the brain takes over so that you can become completely present and peaceful during the meditation. As a result, the left brain is quieted.

The Difference Between the Brain and the Mind

The brain is the physical organ with the two halves explained above. The mind, however, is something completely different. The mind is the observer of how we perceive and think about ourselves, and the world around us.

The extraordinary thing about the mind is consciousness. It is the awareness to observe our thoughts and beliefs and questioning them.

Initially, not everyone understands that we are not our thoughts. Instead, we are the observer of the thoughts. We are not our beliefs. We are the consciousness that observes those beliefs.

When you understand this simple distinction, it opens up possibilities. If we are not our thoughts, and we are the observer of the thoughts, then we actually have power over the thoughts that we think. When we practice thoughts repeatedly, they become beliefs. So if we are not our beliefs and we are not our thoughts, then we have power to choose different thoughts and practice these thoughts to create new beliefs.

Why would you want to choose different thoughts and beliefs? Because our thoughts and beliefs affect the actions we take each day, which in turn, affect our results. Our thoughts end up becoming our reality.

This is a powerful secret that not many people realize. Of the 6000+ thoughts we have each day, most of them are recycled from the past, and most of them are not actually helpful for creating the life that we want.

This is what was happening to me. I was so focused on negative thoughts while I was sick with shingles that it perpetuated more negative thoughts. This then created negative beliefs like how I was a victim of my diagnosis. My actions reflected this way of thinking and my beliefs. I blamed the diagnosis for everything, even things that didn't really relate to shingles like my poor relationships or my business not being as successful as I wanted. And of course, my reality reflected these same things back to me. Lack of success, lack of good relationships, more negative things to focus on. And so, the cycle continued. It was a self-fulfilling prophecy.

While our thoughts can become a loop of negativity, it can just as easily become a loop of positivity too.

This might sound juvenile, commonplace, or even hokey to the reader, but I assure you, when you understand this next concept, everything in your life can change. This is the power of the mind.

The Power of the Mind

The mind is the observer of the thoughts and we have power over what thoughts we want to think daily. Once we start realizing that we can actually choose the thoughts we have each day, then we start believing different things and as a direct consequence, our actions become different too. This ends up changing our results or our external reality.

To put it simply, our mind is the controlling force behind our actions. We just need to wake up to the possibility that we are not yet using our minds to think the best thoughts for us to create the life that we ultimately want.

In order for me to stop my negative thought loop, I needed to first become aware of the negative thoughts. Then once I had recognized these negative thoughts and realized that they were not helping me to create a better life for myself, I then needed to choose more positive and productive thoughts.

At first, it does feel uncomfortable to choose new thoughts. This is because the old thoughts have been deeply ingrained in my mind. But it is possible for these new thoughts to become just as deeply ingrained with practice and repetition. Taking these new thoughts and choosing to think them time and time again is a practice. It takes effort. It will not come easily at first. But after some time, the new thoughts will become the new norm and these will become your new beliefs, which will affect your actions and then your results.

These negative thought loops are one of the things I notice most in people who are trying to eat healthier and/or lose weight. They have been thinking so many negative and degrading thoughts that are actually keeping them stuck and not losing weight.

For instance, I had a client who had been struggling to lose weight. She told me that she had tried everything to lose weight, every diet you could think of. She explained to me what she had been eating, which was relatively clean, but the most important factor that she had not addressed yet was her mindset.

I noticed that she kept thinking to herself:

"I'm never gonna lose the weight. The scale never moves. I am terrible at this. I'm awful. Nothing I do ever matters and I never lose weight."

Imagine if you were thinking these thoughts too on repeat every single day. How does it make you feel about yourself?

You would likely feel unmotivated and not energized to make positive changes to your way of living and you would probably be more inclined to think poorly about your body and food choices too.

So, if she is thinking these thoughts, and not feeling great about herself, the likelihood that she makes healthier food choices actually lowers, which means that she doesn't choose healthier foods and it likely affects other habits, like exercise or getting quality sleep and reducing stress. Thus, she continues to keep the weight on. This is because she has practiced these negative thoughts, which have become beliefs, which then influenced her actions and then her results. She had created her own self-fulfilling prophecy.

The first thing that we started working on was her mindset in relation to her health. We worked on recognizing the negative thought model that she was using and practicing each day. Next, we developed more positive and productive thoughts that would help to reprogram her way of thinking, and in turn, change her daily actions. She started practicing this way of thinking, and she started rewiring her neural pathways, developing new beliefs which affected her actions and her results.

After about forty-five days, she messaged me saying she has just done new measurements on her body. She had lost a total of three inches on her body and her weight was reducing too!

Everything starts with a thought so be mindful about what you are thinking and you will create a new reality for yourself. This conscious awareness of your thoughts is a practice you do every day. Commit to this and you will see transformation.

This is the first step to healing your mind.

➡ Action Items

Take time to answer the following questions honestly and completely in your journal.

* What are your negative thoughts? This can be about anything, and I would recommend for you to focus on your health and wellness first. Allow yourself to write whatever negative thoughts come to mind and not judge yourself on it at all. Just let the writing happen freely.

* Are these thoughts true? Are they really helping you to reach your health and wellness goals?

* If not, what would be more positive and productive thoughts to have instead? Write down all the different positive and productive thoughts you can think of.

* Choose one of the new positive and productive thoughts that you feel a strong emotional connection to, a thought that you can really get behind! Write this new thought down on a Post-it note that you will see frequently throughout the day, or set it up as a reminder on your phone. I suggest seeing/reading/

saying this new thought at least five times a day to start to embed it into your mind. As I mentioned, it may feel strange and like hard work to rewire your brain with a new positive and productive thought, but soon it will become second nature.

The Compounding Effect of Stress

Stress. We have all heard how stress has a huge negative impact on our bodies. But, even I, as a health professional, thought that I was immune to these impacts. I mean, I ate well each day and meditated—shouldn't that be enough?

Turns out, it was not.

I truly believe that stress was the major driving force behind why I had shingles. I did not realize how much stress I was under, but not only that. I didn't realize how much stress my body was holding onto.

Ever since becoming a parent, I had gotten so used to a certain level of stress each day. I didn't notice when that stress level continued to rise gradually, as I took on more responsibilities at work and at home—starting my own business, the pressure to keep up with so-cial events, catching up with friends and family, making sure the laundry was done, sending the kids to school with the required money/toys/books, etc. The list of responsibilities, and thus the stress, kept growing.

When our bodies are stressed, we go into a fight-or-flight mode. We literally force our bodies and minds to make decisions for our survival. This reactionary mode was helpful when we were run-ning away from saber-tooth tigers or away from avalanches and mudslides, but in today's day and age, we usually don't have those types of experiences.

However, our bodies do not know the difference between stress from carnivorous animals and the stress from paying bills on time. So whatever stress we are experiencing, our body still moves into a fight-or-flight mode. Any kind of stress—whether it be from work, family, money, arguments with loved ones, even road rage—can trigger this reactionary response.

We have also been conditioned by society to hold onto that stress and not have enough ways of releasing the pent-up energy that is often associated with stress. Instead, we just keep it to ourselves and find ways to muscle through the tension, frustration and overwhelm. When we do not have sufficient stress relief methods, our body holds onto the stress long after the stressful event has occurred.

The problem is that we don't even realize that our bodies are still under stress and we continue to pile up more and more stress onto ourselves without ever having dealt with the stress from previous weeks, months, or even years.

I knew that I had stress in my life. That is why I started doing stress mitigation techniques, such as meditation, breathwork exercises and journaling. These techniques can be really helpful and powerful, and they worked for me for a long time.

However, these techniques were only treating the symptoms of stress. They helped me to release the stress in my shoulders and gave me temporary relief from the everyday stresses of life.

What I wasn't doing was getting to the reason why I was having stress.

Without getting to the root cause of the stress in my life, I was simply adding more and more stress to my body and mind every single day and not actually releasing the stress through positive and healthy means, then hoping that meditation and breathwork would be the band-aid over the stress that would get me through until the next day.

And at a certain point, that band-aid was no longer working.

I had to make a massive shift in how I was dealing with stress.

The Effect of Stress on the Energetic Body

Stress can have a surprising and detrimental effect on the body. Different people experience different stress responses such as stomach upset (more on this later), headaches, rashes, itching, heart palpitations, etc.

But another stress response I want to share with you is the effect of stress on the energetic body.

The energetic body is a term I use to describe the energy flow throughout the body. We are all energetic beings and energy runs through our energetic centers or chakras. This energy may not be discernible to most human eyes, but you may have felt energy move through you when you walk into a room filled with a huge fun party happening and you instantly feel energized and upbeat. Or you may have felt a weight on your shoulders when you have done something that made you feel guilty, like lying to a loved one.

Our energetic bodies are affected by our environment—aka the situation happening around us—but it can also be affected by what is going on inside of us, aka our thoughts and beliefs.

When we experience prolonged stress, either external or internal, it causes the energetic body to become blocked in certain areas, restricting or stopping the much-needed flow of energy. We can feel unexplainable weight or pressure in certain areas of the body, or have a nagging pain that just won't go away. These are all signs that energy flow is being blocked or stagnated.

A stressed-out body is a body that fights change. Why? Because the body is in that protective mode, otherwise known as the fight mode from the fight-or-flight behaviors explained above. Say, for example, you are desperately trying to lose weight, but you are stressing out about weight loss every single day of your life. You wake up wondering if you've lost any weight overnight, you obsess about portion sizes, what foods are bad foods, how many hours of exercise you do each day, etc. You are in fact piling more and more stress onto your already stressed-out body.

When the physical body experiences this amount of stress for a long period of time, the body itself holds onto weight as a way of protecting itself from change. This makes it so much more difficult to lose weight. There is a branch of science called embodied cognition[8] that looks at the effect of mental states, such as guilt and shame, on how we perceive weight and the feeling of weight on our bodies. Studies have analyzed that when someone feels immense guilt, the individual feels an increased sense of weight in their body. This is literally the embodiment of the feeling of guilt or shame as weight. So now imagine, if you have that feeling for months or years. How would your body feel? The amount of weight that you hold onto, the feeling of the weight on your shoulders, would be tremendous. And, unfortunately, the more that we think those thoughts, the more we feel this weight, and the more the body fights to protect itself, making it a long battle with weight loss.

The Effect of Stress on the Physical Body

Stress can affect all major organs and physical body functions[9].

Stress can impact your hunger levels. Some people may experience either an increased or decreased level of hunger as a result of stress on their bodies.

Stress can also impact the function of your gastrointestinal tract. You may experience changes in how well your GI tract moves food through the intestines, how your gut absorbs the nutrients from food, how permeable the gut lining is, the mucus and stomach acid may be altered, and you may even experience reactivation of previous inflammation in the gut. People with Crohn's disease or ulcerative-based diseases may have more pain, discomfort, or issues with their conditions when their stress levels are heightened.

Stress can reduce the speed of stomach emptying and can increase the colonic motility. When there isn't complete and frequent emptying of the gastrointestinal tract, there is potential for toxins to be reabsorbed into the body. This can have a massive impact on hormone levels as well as toxin levels within the body.

The endocrine system is the system that connects the brain and spinal cord down to the base of your spine. Stress can affect the endocrine system in either negative or positive ways. Most notably, the hypothalamic-pituitary-adrenal axis can be greatly negatively affected by prolonged stress.

When we obsess about weight loss, speaking physiologically now, the additional stress on our bodies actually causes increased inflammation in the body, which can exacerbate existing issues like digestive problems, hormonal imbalances, issues recognizing hunger and fullness cues, increased gut microbiome issues, etc. When stress is prolonged in the body, it has not only been linked to greater weight gain or difficulty in losing weight, but also many chronic diseases like high blood pressure, diabetes, Irritable Bowel Syndrome and many others[10]. This chronic inflammation and even chronic stress have been called the Silent Killer because it can often occur without you even realizing it and can be very challenging to address and release without great awareness and purposeful consistent action.

The Effect of Stress on the Brain and Gut Health

Just in case the possibility of getting shingles due to stress wasn't enough to cause you to look into your own stress levels, let me tell you about what happens when the gut is stressed for a long amount of time and how it impacts your brain health specifically.

Prolonged psychological stress has been linked to a heightened risk of depression[11], which can also impact your gut health. This is because of something called the Gut-Brain Axis. This is a channel that works in two directions, meaning that anything affecting the gut can then have an impact on brain health, and conversely, anything affecting the brain can have an impact on gut health.

When we experience stress, our autonomic nervous system and circulatory system carry distress signals to the gut. This causes a restriction in blood flow to the gut lining. This stress triggers pathogenic bacteria to be produced, causing dysbiosis and leaky gut, two conditions attributed to poor gut health. Dysbiosis is simply the imbalance of bad bacteria in the gut vs good bacteria. Leaky gut is the term for when the cells in the gut lining have become porous and permeable, which allows for toxins and food particles to enter the bloodstream as opposed to getting eliminated through the gastrointestinal tract. Both dysbiosis and leaky gut syndrome increase inflammation in the body.

In fact, symptoms such as constipation, diarrhea, intense pain in your digestive tract, pain when trying to pass stool or during digestion, bloating, gassiness, etc may be signs of leaky gut or dysbiosis. Inability to eliminate stool from the body can also cause reabsorption of certain toxins, causing them to stay in our bodies, causing more stress on our organs and cells and impacting our wellbeing.

The alteration in the balance of good and bad gut bacteria can cause changes in stress hormone production, inflammation and produce more metabolites, toxins and neurohormones that can affect your mood and what you feel like eating. Changes in gut bacteria may even affect reward pathways in the brain, how your appetite-modulating vagus nerve acts, your taste receptors, and even your appetite levels. One study of two groups of women had half the women drinking a sugar-sweetened drink three times a day for two weeks, while the other group had an aspartame-sweetened drink instead. After two weeks, scientists found that stressed individuals preferentially consumed sugar and increased fat intake enhanced stress reactivity.

One commonly prescribed medication is antibiotics. While antibiotics can be helpful for some, it may also be useful to know the potential negative impact on your gut health from using antibiotics, especially multiple doses. One large study from the UK showed that antibiotics use actually increased the risk of anxiety or depression[12] by about 20%, while multiple courses of antibiotics increase the risk by up to 50%. Not only that, antibiotics cannot differentiate between the good and bad gut bacteria. They end up killing both types of bacteria, which then can impact your gut health too.

Stress can affect both your food choices and how your metabolism works. Increased stress can cause your metabolic rate to lower, meaning you burn less calories and the potential for gaining weight increases.

I often ignored signs of stress and thought that just having a massage every other week was enough to reduce my stress levels. Boy, was I wrong. Stress puts the body into survival mode—a fight-or-flight state—literally forcing the body to do something in order to survive. Little did I realize that I had been putting my body into survival mode for months, if not years. The stress reduction strategies I was doing were helping a little, but the ultimate way to reduce stress is to confront and then release the causes of stress, not just fight the symptoms of stress. I committed to reducing any and all stress, as much as humanly possible. I also combined this with getting more sleep (see Step 4 in Part one above) in order to reduce my stress hormone levels. This was a practice that I did for over several months, even though my shingles rash had decreased after about ten days. I was finally able to see what a huge impact stress was having on my body, and how important stress management and sleep were to mitigating this.

How to Find the Root Cause of Your Stress

Finding the root cause to your stress is key to releasing and reducing the stress in your life. Here are my three simple steps to finding the real reasons for your stress.

Step 1: Determine what events/people cause you to feel stress

You may have already had something or someone pop into your head that is the reason for your stress. And if you do, that is great awareness!

But if you don't know exactly what is causing your stress, here is a simple exercise you can try in order to figure it out.

At the beginning of the day in your day planner or schedule, write down all the meetings and activities you have planned. Then as the day progresses, write down your stress level on a scale of 1-10, one being no stress at all and ten being major high stress. You can also write down what about that meeting or activity caused you stress, e.g. boss was yelling at me, I missed a huge mistake in a report, had a fight with my spouse, kids not listening to me, etc. Here is an example table you can use to guide you:

Date

Time	Task	Stress Triggers	Stress Level (1-10)
6 am			
7 am			
8 am			
9 am			
10 am			
11 am			
12 noon			
1 pm			
2 pm			
3 pm			
4 pm			
5 pm			
6 pm			
7 pm			
8 pm			
9 pm			
10 pm			

You can repeat this exercise as long as it takes for you to begin to see a trend. Do you notice that your ranking of stress is higher at work or home? Are you having high stress with one particular person or event?

These are all great clues as to what in your life is causing you the most stress. You may have one main cause or several. Accept what is and then let's move to how you can release this stress.

Step 2: Find ways to mitigate your stress

The next step is asking yourself what you can do to reduce stress in this area of life. Here are some ideas:

* Minimizing interactions with that person causing you stress

* Declining superfluous meetings as much as possible

* Requesting to be transferred out of toxic, stressful teams

* Having difficult conversations that you have been putting off

* Establishing boundaries with people who are impinging on yours

* Carpooling with a friend if driving in rush hour traffic causes you stress

* Extending any deadlines to give you more time to complete work

* Taking projects off your plate and delegating them or postponing them to a later time

* Stop committing to things you don't actually want to do just because your mother/sister/spouse/friend etc wants you to do them

Of course, these are just a few ideas to get you started. There are more stress mitigation techniques coming up in the next section too. But it is truly up to you to find solutions to the stress problems in your life. It may seem challenging at first, but I assure you it will be worth it in the long run so that your stress levels are greatly reduced and your health is greatly improved.

Step 3: Review how well the stress mitigation techniques are working

After you have tried your stress reduction techniques for a week or two, reflect and see how well this technique has worked. Spending just five minutes to check in and see if you still would rank your stress levels at the same number on the scale of 1-10 can be very helpful to see if your stress is reducing or if you need to try a different approach.

Effective Stress Mitigation Techniques

Now that we know more about the effect of stress on our physiological and energetic bodies, now it is time to learn about various stress mitigation techniques.

The following are some of my favorite stress mitigation techniques. I would suggest trying these in conjunction with trying to reduce the causes of stress as much as possible. I've also included some great resources and simple instructions for each of these techniques.

Sleep

Sleep is one of the most powerful ways to allow your body and mind to relax and release the tension of the day.

Experts recommend aiming for at least 7–9 hours of sleep per night. During sleep, the brain sorts and processes the day, moving short-term memories to long-term memories. The pituitary gland in the brain releases growth hormone so that the body can repair itself. Your cortisol levels reduce, blood pressure lowers, your immune system is boosted and your sympathetic nervous system – which controls the fight or flight response – can relax.

If you'd like to improve the duration or quality of your sleep, try some of these tips:

* Aim to stop eating heavy foods or drinking caffeine several hours before your bedtime. Having a very full belly can cause discomfort which may prevent you from sleeping. Caffeine affects individuals differently, so if you are sensitive to caffeine you may want to keep caffeine drinks to the morning time. Lastly, alcohol may make it easier for you to fall asleep, however, studies have shown that alcohol does reduce the quality of sleep.

* Have a wind-down routine prior to bedtime e.g. brushing your teeth, washing your face, gentle stretching, and/or reading, etc. This routine can include as few or as many steps as you would like. The key is to do it consistently so that your body starts to connect this routine with getting ready for sleep. Ideally, ensure your routine helps you to slow down, relax and get your mind and body ready for sleep.

* Aim to stop screen usage at least one hour prior to bedtime. The blue light from screens can interfere with your circadian rhythm which impacts your ability to fall asleep and stay asleep.

* Make your bedroom a cool and dark place to help make sleeping easier. Thick curtains to block out light and a fan or setting the AC to a comfortable and cool temperature can be helpful for this.

* Keep a notepad by your bedside to write down any thoughts or to-do's that might pop up as you're preparing to sleep. This helps to get the list of tasks out of your head, while knowing that you will remember to look at that list the following day.

Meditation

Many people think that meditation is sitting cross-legged on the floor saying "Om" repeatedly. This is one method of meditation, but there are many other methods as well.

People often think that meditation involves completely clearing the mind and having no thoughts. But in actuality, meditation is becoming the gentle observer to the thoughts that occur and lovingly release them to focus on a specific topic or way of being.

The benefit of meditation is that it allows you to find the moment of pause between a situation occurring and how you respond to it. We often get blindsided by something happening in our lives so we jump across the table at someone, or rush out the door, or get into arguments, etc without having properly allowed ourselves to think and process the situation. When you start understanding that you don't have to just react to situations, that you get to have a mindful response, this totally changes how you interact with people, and how they interact with you.

Meditation allows us to get deeply in tune with our thoughts and actions so that we can continue to bring that same mindfulness to all areas of our lives.

Here are a few ways you can get started with meditation if you're a beginner:

Guided Meditations

One of the easiest ways to get started with meditation is to find a five-minute guided meditation on Youtube. A guided meditation is where someone is speaking and walking you through a specific visualization. I recommend starting the meditation by sitting in a comfortable chair, laying down on a bed or floor, or sitting on the floor with your back against the wall. Play the guided meditation and just allow yourself to listen and let your imagination follow the guidance.

Observe your thoughts and visualization without judgment. I have listed some resources for quick meditations here: http://www. nourishwithrenata.com/healyourbodymindandspirit

Non-guided Meditations

These meditations use music or sounds only in the videos. There is no speaking. Sometimes the music is a simple instrumental piece, or the video may use Tibetan singing bowls, or any single instrument to create the mood for the meditation. The music may swell during the meditation to help guide you throughout the meditation process.

Mantras in Meditations

There may be a mantra, or saying, that you want to repeat to yourself during the meditation. Mantras can be very useful to help to keep your mind focused on meditation, as opposed to wayward thoughts popping up into your mind all the time. Some examples of mantras that you can use during meditation are:

* I am peaceful

* I am worthy

* I am loved

* I am whole

You can also create your own mantras based on something that you are focusing on at the time.

The 5 Senses Meditation

This type of meditation can be very easy to do, especially if you're not in a quiet place. This meditation allows you to become engrossed in the current moment because you purposefully activate your awareness to each of the five senses.

✻ Start by taking three deep breaths, allowing the inhale to expand the belly and chest, then fully exhaling to release all the breath, pulling the belly button into the spine.

✻ Now become mindful of what you see. Name what you see with simple one-word nouns e.g. tree, grass, pavement, dog, man, etc.

✻ Become mindful of what you hear. Name what you hear e.g. wind, rustling, birds, traffic, etc.

✻ Become mindful of what you feel. Name them e.g. the wind, sun, clothes, bracelet, watch, etc.

✻ Become mindful of what you smell. Name what you smell e.g. flowers, grass, air freshener, etc.

✻ Become mindful of what you taste. Name it e.g. water, saliva, coffee remnants, tea remnants, food, etc.

✻ Continue cycling through the senses, or spend extra time in each of these senses until your allocated meditation time is completed, or you feel calmer and more relaxed.

Walking Meditations

Sometimes sitting still for a meditation can be uncomfortable for those people that like to move around, so a slow walking meditation can be very helpful for this. While out for a walk in nature, allow yourself to become very mindful of each breath, focusing deeply on each inhale and exhale.

How does the breath feel as you inhale and exhale? Follow the breath as it comes in and out. Notice how the air feels as the breath enters the nose, then as it exits. Become fully engrossed in the feeling of the breath.

Now focus on each step you are taking. Notice how the heel of your foot presses down against the ground and rocks forward till the toes press into the earth and lift. Notice the other foot doing the same thing, but there is overlap of when the heel hits the ground vs when the other toes lift. Really immerse yourself in the walking movement.

Journaling

For a long time, I had some resistance to journaling. It felt like it would be a lot of work to write things down and then there was the fear of someone finding what I had journaled and then getting upset about it.

If you think that journaling will be a lot of work, firstly, don't even worry about using a hardcover journal and pen. Simply use the Notes app on your phone or a Word or Google doc. You can password protect most online documents so this helps to prevent anyone from finding it.

To get started with journaling, set a timer for literally just five minutes and let yourself write whatever you want. Don't think about it—just write! Also, you don't have to read back what you write at all. Just allow the words to flow and be released from your body without judgment and without needing to justify it to yourself.

As time goes on, you may recognize that journaling in this way, or even for longer periods of time, is actually quite cathartic. It is a method of releasing your thoughts and feelings without having to need someone else to listen to you or feel afraid of how to say something without jeopardizing relationships or incurring judgment. I truly believe that journaling is a powerful method for working through thoughts and feelings, as well as releasing pent-up frustrations and emotions without harboring anyone else with those thoughts.

Lastly, if you are really worried about someone finding your journal notes, rip out the pages of your journal, and safely burn them. You can do this outside in a fireproof pot, in a firepit, or even on your stove with a source of extinguishing any runaway fires at close proximity. Burning your journal notes is another method of releasing and has distinct finality to the release. Once it is burned, it is gone forever, both physically and emotionally.

If you're not sure where to get started with journaling, here are three ideas that can help you begin.

1. **Five-minute journaling:** Set a timer for five minutes and write down what has been troubling you or something that has been on your mind. Let yourself write anything and everything that comes to mind. It may be helpful to ask yourself questions like:

   a. Why is this important to me?

   b. Why is this bothering me?

   c. What emotions is this situation bringing up?

   d. What am I afraid will happen in this situation?

2. **Journal prompts:** To get you started journaling, especially if you are feeling stuck, use the following prompts to start the writing process:

   a. Today, something that bothered me was…

   b. I am feeling _____ because_____

   c. Today was a _____ (good/bad/frustrating/peaceful) day because _____

   d. I am stressed out because_____

   e. I really wish that _____ would be/do/act like this _____

3. **Free writing:** The process of free writing is similar to the first point. If you would like to write for a particular timeframe, set a timer. Alternatively, you may set yourself up in your favorite room of the house where you will not be interrupted. Taking your favorite journal and pen, or even the Notes app on your phone, allow yourself to write literally anything that comes to mind. You can even write random words or blah blah blah, if you want, to get you started. After a few seconds, you will find that your mind will start to bring up thoughts that you will feel pulled to write about. Explain the thoughts that come to mind, write down the feelings that you're experiencing. Get everything off your chest. Ideally keep writing nonstop and don't even think about spelling or grammar. Let the pen fly across the page until you feel completely spent, or until all of the thoughts and energy around that particular situation are all written down. You don't have to reread your journal entries if you don't want to. You can discard the pages by burning, shredding, or throwing them away if that is what you prefer. The key with free writing is to write with abandon, totally allowing your thoughts and feelings to be expressed on paper without worry or concern over the outcome. It is a powerful way of releasing thoughts and feelings from the subconscious mind, that you may not have taken the time to acknowledge and become aware of in your conscious mind.

Breathwork

I discovered breathwork a few years ago and could not possibly tout the benefits more. We all breathe without really realizing it every day as we go about our daily actions. But because it is such an automatic body function, we forget that paying attention to our breath can actually help us to relieve stress, relax, and even cultivate a deeper connection with spirit.

Scientifically speaking, the benefits of purposeful and mindful breathing practices are attributed to a chemical called DMT or N-Dimethyltryptamine. This is a psychedelic drug found in plants like ayahuasca and in animals[13], including humans. However, research in the 1950s and 60s suggested that DMT is synthesized in the lungs and pineal gland in the brain. The pineal gland is often associated with the Third Eye chakra (more on this in Section three), which affects visualization. As a result, people believe that during meditation and purposeful deep breathing exercises, where the lungs are being used to a greater capacity, DMT is also produced in greater amounts, which can affect what you visualize or see during these practices. This is often called an altered state or is connected with a spiritual experience, such as seeing visions, guidance, etc. Now, don't be scared that trying out meditation or breathwork is going to cause you to have hallucinations like you are taking drugs. In fact, some people do not experience any altered states of being while doing these activities and simply experience reduced stress and tension.

Conversely, there are some people that do experience the effect of DMT or a DMT-type situation. There does not appear to be enough scientific evidence to explain this fully, but the brain is a complex organ and we don't understand much about how the brain works or why it does what it does during certain situations. Some researchers believe that DMT may trigger the imagination more than the rational mind which leads to altered states of being or visualizations. The enzyme and gene that synthesize DMT are active in the retina too, so this explains why seeing visions is a potential when DMT is increased. Some spiritual people liken this to reaching states of enlightenment or experience guidance from the Divine or some other higher power.

While research is still limited in this area, what I know is only from my own experience. There have definitely been times in meditation or deep, purposeful breathing practices that I have seen visions in my mind's eye or I have received guidance on a question I had had in my mind for a while. Whether this came from increased DMT produced by my body, or an active imagination, or even being consciously aware of what I was seeing as I was in a state between being awake and being asleep, I will never know. But what I do know is that breathwork has helped me tremendously to de-stress, relax, regroup, recharge and to be reassured when I was searching for guidance or answers to my questions on my path, my future and my purpose.

Getting started with breathwork is as easy as becoming mindful and purposeful with your breathing practices. Below you will find three easy breathwork practices to help you get started today.

Breathwork Practice 1: Observing Your Natural Breathing Pattern

The essential starting point of breathwork is to become the gentle observer of your natural breathing pattern. Read the following steps, and also find the follow-along video at: http://www.nourishwithrenata.com/healyourbodymindandspirit

* Start by sitting in a comfortable position, either in a high-backed chair, against a wall, or cross-legged on the floor.

* Aim to have your back straight, head above heart, and heart above pelvis. We want your spine to be fully aligned and comfortable without any additional tension or stress on the body.

* Place your hands on your lap, palms facing upwards if possible or in whatever position feels right to you.

* Gently close your eyes or gaze down at the floor at a point that is unmoving.

* Breathe as naturally as possible and just notice the breath as it moves in and out of your nose.

* After a few breaths, shift your focus to the rise and fall of your chest as you breathe. Notice the rise or inhale, the brief pause, then the fall on the exhale, before another brief pause. Try not to control the breath and simply notice the inhales and exhales.

* If a thought enters your mind, allow yourself to notice the thought, then come back to the breath. It is totally normal to become distracted during the first several attempts at breathwork. This is because your mind is used to being overly stimulated and jumping from one exciting thought to the next. Comparatively, focusing on your breathing is not as exciting as many other things. But keep coming back to your breath. Focus on the inhales and exhales. Focus on allowing the breath, being that gentle observer and not controlling. Just notice.

If you are ready for the next step, you can begin focusing on any areas of the body that may be holding tension.

* Notice your shoulders. Are they hunched upwards towards your ears? If so, imagine that you are breathing into the shoulders and with each exhale, you are allowing that tension in your shoulders to melt away, releasing your shoulders down and removing any tension.

* Notice your jaw. Are you clenching or tightening your jaw? If so, imagine you are breathing into the jaw now. Allow each exhale to release tension and the clenching feeling from the jaw, melting any tension down and away from the jaw until it is completely relaxed.

Continue with this process of finding any areas in the body that feel stressed. Areas you can focus on include the forehead, the back, the chest, the legs, the hands, or anywhere else that you become aware that you are holding tension. The key is to continue to breathe into those areas. Let the inhales bring in calmness and let the exhales release any tension in the muscles.

Repeat this practice for 5-10 minutes or work up to these times if need be. This, like anything else, is a practice so you may need multiple attempts until you feel comfortable doing this or even feel somewhat relaxed afterwards.

I recommend doing this or some form of breathwork practice daily as a stress mitigation practice.

Breathwork Practice 2: Diaphragmatic Breathing

Many of us are breathing in a shallow manner, as in not breathing as deeply as we could be. This is because we have been conditioned to be very self-conscious about our stomach regions and often spend much of the day sucking in the stomach to appear thinner or smaller. Instead with this practice, I want you to start releasing this conditioning because we are going to learn how to breathe into the diaphragm.

The diaphragm is a muscle that sits below the lungs at the base of the chest. It separates the abdomen from the chest. It is shaped like a dome and it contracts continually and generally involuntarily. When we inhale, the diaphragm contracts and moves downwards in the chest, creating more space in the chest for the lungs to expand. When we exhale, the lungs minimize, the diaphragm relaxes and moves upward in the chest. However, what we are going to learn is to breathe all the way into the diaphragm instead of simply breathing into the chest, which is what most people do. If you've ever noticed your breath quickening in stressful situations, you are breathing into the chest only. The alternative is to breathe deeply down into the belly or diaphragm.

Consciously breathing into the diaphragm, also known as diaphragmatic breathing, abdominal breathing or belly breathing, encourages full oxygen exchange meaning that there is more complete trade of the oxygen entering the body, with the carbon dioxide leaving the body. Because of this, the heartbeat and blood pressure can lower or stabilize, giving that feeling of tension or stress relief and a greater sense of relaxation.

Diaphragmatic breathing stimulates the vagus nerve, a nerve that runs from the belly, all the way up the back of the neck and to the brain. This stimulation activates the parasympathetic nervous system, otherwise known as the rest and digest nervous system. This allows us to begin or continue the feeling of relaxation associated with this breathing practice.

For the following breathwork practice, read through and follow the steps below, or see the video at: http://www.nourishwithrenata. com/healyourbodymindandspirit

* Start in a comfortable position, seated on a chair, against a wall or cross legged on the ground.

* Ensure your head is above your heart, which is above your pelvis. Once again, we are looking for comfortable spinal alignment.

* You may find it helpful to close your eyes to be able to connect with the feeling of the chest or the belly filling with air as the practice continues. Alternatively, you may find it easier to look into a mirror while you do this practice until you become more comfortable with it.

✳ Place your hands on your chest, roughly in the middle where your heart is.

✳ Allow yourself to become the gentle observer of your breath. Notice if your hands rise and fall as you inhale and exhale. Typically, this will happen first and is easier to feel or see as it occurs. You are breathing into your chest, so on the inhale, your chest lifts, and on the exhale, your chest falls. This is how most people breathe on a day-to-day basis. Notice the movement of the chest, notice the inhales and exhales. Once you are comfortable with this, move onto the next step.

✳ Gently shift your hands to rest on your belly. Begin to notice if the belly is moving as you breathe. Most people will not notice a big change in the belly moving at first. This is totally ok.

Now we will begin to learn how to breathe diaphragmatically.

✳ On your next inhale, imagine that your body is a vase and the breath is water that you are pouring from the top of the vase (your nose and mouth) into the bottom of the vase (your belly). The "water," or breath, will travel all the way down to the belly to fill up the "vase." You may notice the belly start to expand on the inhale. As it does so, your hands on your belly will lift also. This is good. You are breathing into the diaphragm.

✳ On the exhale, gently pull the belly button towards the spine and notice the belly fall. The hands on the belly will fall also. Empty your vase.

✳ Continue with this visualization, if it is helpful, or simply begin to inhale down to the belly. Notice your hands on your belly lifting with the inhale, then exhaling as your belly and your hands fall.

* This is the practice of diaphragmatic breathing. It is very soothing and calming to breathe this deeply and this purposefully.

* Continue with this practice for five minutes or even up to an hour if you have the time and have been gradually working up to this practice.

It is possible that you may experience dizziness, tingly sensations through the body, pins-and-needles sensations in the hands and feet, etc. This is actually quite normal, although it can be quite unnerving at times. If you start feeling very disoriented or imbalanced, it may be helpful to lie down during this practice or, as mentioned, gradually work at increasing the amount of time that you can do this diaphragmatic breathing.

To finish the practice, I recommend doing one to three breath holds. To do this, take a deep inhale down to the diaphragm, then hold the breath. Try not to clench or add additional tension to the body as you hold the breath for as long as you can. You may be surprised at how long you can hold your breath for. Then when you are ready, gently release the breath through the mouth. Breathe in your natural breathing pattern for a few breaths, then repeat the breath holds as desired.

Note, it is not recommended for women during the bleed phase of their menstrual cycles to do breath holds because it adds additional tension to the pelvic floor, which may already be under pain or increased stress during this time. Of course, you are the best advocate for your body, and you have full responsibility and control over your breathwork practice, no matter what phase of your cycle you are in.

Breathwork Practice 3: Alternate Nostril Breathing

Alternate nostril breathing, also known as Nadi Shodhana Pranayama, is a yogic breathing practice. Some say that alternate nostril breathing can help with opening up both sides of the brain. A 2016 scientific study looked at the contralateral frontal hemodynamics[14], or the activation of different sides of the brain, when doing alternate nostril breathing. It found that there are measurable cognitive changes, including increased oxygenation and blood volume, that are induced by the alternate nostril breathing technique.

I've created a free video to show how to do alternate nostril breathing that you can see at http://www.nourishwithrenata.com/healyourbodymindandspirit

Here are the steps to do this method:

* Sit in a comfortable position, either in a chair, against a wall, or cross-legged on the floor.

* If it is helpful, you can roll your shoulders or neck to start to relax and settle into the breathwork practice.

* You can begin by taking three deep inhales and exhales, breathing deep into the diaphragm, holding the inhale for a second or two, then fully exhaling by drawing the belly button into the spine. Repeat this for a total of three deep inhales and exhales.

* Now we will begin learning how to do the alternate nostril breathing pattern.

* Take your right hand and gently press the right nostril down using the right thumb.

* Inhale through the left nostril. Pause.

* Exhale through the left nostril.

* Take your right ring finger and gently press on the left nostril to close it. Pause with both nostrils closed for a second. Lift the right thumb to open the right nostril.

* Inhale through the right nostril. Pause.

* Exhale through the right nostril. Pause.

* Close the right nostril with the right thumb. Pause with both nostrils closed for a second.

* Lift the right ring finger to open the left nostril.

* Inhale through the left nostril. Pause.

* Exhale through the left nostril. Pause. Close the left nostril with the right ring finger. Pause with both nostrils closed. Lift the right thumb to open the right nostril.

Repeat this process of closing off one nostril at a time and allowing a full inhale, pause, exhale, and then pause before closing the other nostril.

You can do this alternative breathing practice for five minutes and work your way up to ten minutes or more, depending on how much you enjoy the practice.

To finish the practice, remove your right hand from your face and move into your natural breathing pattern. Notice how the nostrils, the face, the body all feel different after this practice. How does your mind feel? Do you notice any changes? For me, it is almost as if I notice that my brain has been oxygenated and is open to much more awareness after performing this practice.

There are many other breathing practices that you can try also. Several breathing practices are available on YouTube and I have also included video demonstrations of all the breathing practices explained above at http://www.nourishwithrenata.com/healyourbodymindandspirit

Ultimately, I have found breathwork to be an incredible healing practice, a tool to help me to uncover and deal with feelings and thoughts that I may have been suppressing, and overall, helping me to release my negative thoughts or limiting beliefs that may be holding me back.

Why Mindfulness Practices are so Important

Breathwork, journaling, and meditation are also known by another name—mindfulness practices. These practices not only have a huge impact to our stress levels, lowering them, and in turn increasing our quality of life, but it affects another key aspect of ourselves—our intuition.

When we have a consistent mindfulness practice, like one of the methods listed above, it allows our left brain to quiet. The right brain then becomes more dominant, allowing us to settle into peace and calm, and find what is often called The Flow. When we experience this quieting of the left brain and more peace from the right brain, it enables us to hear our intuition speak. We are able to hear our inner voice guiding us. The noise of the outside world being filtered through the left brain's chatter often masks or overpowers the inner voice. So, spending more time in quiet, through mindfulness practices can help us tune in and hear what our intuition is telling us more clearly. Unlocking your connection with your intuition can help you heal your body, mind, and spirit.

PART 3

Heal Your Spirit

I didn't consider myself much of a religious or spiritual person for most of my life. It wasn't until I started on my personal development journey—more specifically my health and fitness journey—that I started to see things a little bit differently. I once heard entrepreneur, Lori Harder, explain in a podcast that fitness and nutrition is like the gateway to spiritual growth. When I heard that, I felt like there was no better explanation.

When you start to work on healing your body through food and exercise, it allows you to open up your awareness to a new way of being—a way of being that is possibly unlike what you have ever experienced before. You have an insight and consciousness into how your body is so much more than just a vessel of muscles and tendons. You start to appreciate how your mind can expand and challenge your body to extend itself past the limits that you previously thought. You engage your imagination and visualization to elevate your current circumstances.

After many years of working on my physical and mental awareness, I tapped into the idea of spirituality. Now, this means something different from religion and I am not about to force any particular belief system on you. In this section, all I want to do is open your awareness up to the possibility that beyond physical, mental, and emotional healing, there is another level: spirituality.

Spirituality can mean different things to different people. When I refer to spirituality, I am referring to a belief that there is something greater than us human beings, such as God for some people, the Universe for others. The word Source is often referred to, as well.

This belief of a greater existence above our current human existence can be debated in many ways so if the feeling of skepticism has risen up in you, I accept that. That is a valid feeling that we all have at one time or another. I certainly have! All I ask is for you to be open to the possibility of a deeper healing experience than you may have felt physically, mentally, and emotionally so far in your life.

Alternatively, you may have a spiritual practice that you have been doing regularly, one that has served you well in the past. That is fantastic, and for you, I also ask that you have an open mind to new methodologies or practices to try in your next spiritual routine.

This section on healing your spirit is all about helping you under- stand how your energy and spiritual connection can affect your body and mind, as well as introduce some practices to help deepen your connection with an existence greater than us.

The Disconnect

I believe that many people have a disconnect between their spir- it and their bodies. We are often in such a fast-paced society that we forget that we need to slow down and listen to what our bodies are telling us. If we do not slow down enough to listen, our bodies will eventually find some way of letting us know that something is wrong such as having a medical condition or an emotional or men- tal breakdown. Listening to our bodies is simply another name for the practice of paying attention to your intuition.

What is Intuition?

Intuition is a word that often makes cynics and scientific people cringe. It's a word used by a lot of people who believe in spirituality and energy.

But did you know that there is actually a scientific basis for intuition? Studies have shown that intuition is the subconscious mind's way of processing thousands of pieces of data coming into the brain through our senses. Think of the subconscious mind as a huge computer, taking in so much data and quickly processing it per our request. When we have a decision we want to make, our subconscious mind makes a split-second decision using all of these pieces of data it has. The problem is that our conscious mind cannot keep up with the rate of this decision-making process so it can seem like a magical, pulled-out-of-the-air type of decision, but it is actually based on real information.

In many cases, intuition has been given a bad rap for many years, which can result in us not trusting what our intuition is telling us. I believe this bad rap is because people really didn't understand what intuition was. Thankfully, science is helping to show evidence to these nay-sayers so that we start to trust our intuition again.

And if that wasn't enough evidence for you, I believe many of the professions that we look up to use their intuition, they just call it a different name. Athletes, law enforcement, and mothers talk about a gut feeling, an inner knowing, or a hunch. This is just one way that our intuition speaks to us.

Why is Intuition such a Big Part of Your Healing Journey?

Sigmund Freud, the famed Austrian neurologist and psychoanalyst, was the first person to talk about the three levels of the human brain.

1. **The Conscious Mind:** Awareness of self in space and time; also includes things we know about ourselves and the environment around us.

2. **The Subconscious Mind:** Thoughts that are unconscious at a particular moment but can be recalled as needed, such as memories, to make them conscious.

3. **The Unconscious Mind:** Things outside of our conscious awareness

The human brain can take in over eleven million bits of information every second. This information comes from our senses, such as what we see, hear, feel, etc. The conscious mind only accounts for about forty to fifty bits of information per second, thus our subconscious mind is the part of our brain that is absorbing and processing a huge chunk of the information fed to the brain.

Our subconscious minds are processing so much information about the outside world but also taking in just as much information about our bodies and our health. The subconscious mind is keeping tabs on things like if you're feeling dryness in your mouth, a precursor to dehydration, if you're starting to feel hungry, if you have an ache or pain in one area of the body, etc. In my opinion, our bodies are incredibly wise due to all of the information it takes in and our body is imparting this wisdom to our brains through subtle indications, feelings, and clues. That is why I always say that our bodies are telling us clues all the time. These clues are simply a direct byproduct of all of the sensory data that our subconscious mind has processed and trying to tell the conscious mind to do something about it.

Another name for these clues is your intuition. The amazing thing about intuition is that when we learn to listen to it as well as take action on it, our intuition strengthens. We are also better able to connect deeply with how our body is feeling and what it needs in that moment.

These intuitive hits are a powerful tool to understanding what foods your body needs now. This is different to a craving, which may be influenced by your external environment or people. Your intuition speaks to you from deep within, a knowing, that sense of a sure thing. And when you listen to that intuition and take action or consume the food that your intuition is telling you to eat, that is when you bring together the energetic body, physical body, and mind to have the most healing impact.

How Does Your Intuition Speak To You?

I like to think of intuition as a muscle. The more you use this muscle, the stronger your intuition gets and the more that you trust the information that your intuition tells you.

The first step of strengthening your intuition muscle is to understand how your intuition speaks to you. Do you feel something in the pit of your stomach, a lifting or a dropping feeling telling you yes or no? Do you feel butterflies in your heart or a swelling of energy? Do you have an inner dialogue in your mind that tells you when something is awry?

These are all ways that your intuition can speak to you. I have found that my intuition may speak to me a little differently on different days or during different events in my life. The key is to be open to and aware of how your intuition may be speaking to you.

There are nine ways in which intuition may speak to you. These nine languages are from the book *The Soul's Brain* by Dr Catherine Wilkins. When I read these nine languages, it really helped me understand my own experiences with intuition and how to label it in a way that helps me to develop my intuitive practice.

First of all, your intuition can speak to you either directly or indirectly.

Direct intuition is literal—you may get a sense of exactly what you need to do in a particular situation, like a gut feeling saying I really need to slow down or my life is getting way too out of control.

Indirect intuition is more symbolic. I love this example of an indirect intuitive dream from Charlson Meadows. Imagine you are dreaming that you are at the gym. You get on a treadmill and start running. In the dream, the treadmill begins to speed up, somehow going faster and faster even though you're not touching the speed button. You feel ok with this at first, but you notice continually speeding up your running is starting to get more and more challenging. You start struggling to keep up because the treadmill keeps getting faster. You try to turn off the treadmill but you can't. You keep trying to run faster and faster and faster but it is getting so hard and you can't keep up and then...you wake up. An interpretation of the dream is it being symbolic for your life running out of control and you cannot keep up with it, so the dream is indirectly telling you to start slowing down or soon life will be going too fast for you to keep up.

Here are the nine languages that you may experience with your intuition. One or more of these may resonate with you, depending on the situation.

1: A gut feeling or Clairsentience

This is the most familiar intuitive language because you feel this distinct sensation through your gut or belly. For me, I feel a rising up or a lifting indicating a positive experience or a Yes feeling. Conversely, I may feel a dropping, draining, or lowering feeling that indicates a negative feeling. The term clairsentience is used to describe how your intuition speaks to you through sensory perception.

2: Empathy or intuition through emotion

If you are an empathic person, this means that you can pick up on or get a sense of another person's emotions without them having to tell you or express their emotion to you. Your intuition may use empathy or emotions to indicate a certain issue or feeling about a decision or situation.

3: Hearing thoughts or words aka Clairaudience

Your intuition may speak to you through words that you hear. This doesn't mean that you are hearing voices. It means your intuition is literally speaking to you. You can also think of your intuition as that wise voice from within guiding you with your choices.

4: Hearing sounds as intuition or another form of Clairaudience

Similar to the previous language, this fourth language lends itself to hearing more sounds or tones versus words. These sounds may be symbolic to you or how you are feeling. The key is to figure out how to interpret those sounds in order to gain understanding.

5: Symbols or Clairvisual

Your intuition speaks to you through what you see. It may be seeing in your mind's eye, dreaming or visualizing particular symbols during meditation or just in everyday life. Once again, these symbols are of particular value to you and your experience.

6: Images as intuition or Clairvoyance

This language allows you to see images as if you are watching a movie. It may be memories or almost like an image or visualization of something in the future. It may come to you in a daydream, a sleeping dream, or even in a meditation.

The next three intuitive languages are less common but may be something that you have experienced in the past.

7: Intuition through smell or Clairalience

For some people, their intuition may allow them to smell certain scents that they can interpret to help them with making decisions. This language may act in accordance with another language to add depth to an intuitive hit.

8: Intuition through taste or Clairgustance

Understanding any unexpected tastes on your tongue could be a way that your intuition is speaking to you. You will, of course, have to discern if this is happening from any food you've been eating or drinks you've had previously, but if not, then it could be a fun way your intuition is speaking to you.

And lastly, 9: Intuitive knowing or Claircognizance

That deep, knowing feeling from inside yourself that something is a sure thing. You just know it to be true and there are no two ways about it.

Like I mentioned you may have experienced one or more of these intuitive languages at different times. Moving forward it may be helpful to know the most prominent way that you have felt your intuition speak to you and focus on working that "muscle."

Strengthening Your Intuition

I believe that our bodies are telling us clues all the time about what our body's need. But, like I mentioned before, we often don't even listen to our intuition let alone take action on what our intuition is telling us to do.

Once we become aware of our intuition and how our intuition speaks to you, we can then start practicing listening to our intuition and doing what it says. Every time we do this, we are essentially doing reps to make this muscle bigger and stronger.

There are many exercises that can help you to strengthen your intuition. The following three exercises are impactful and easy to implement. Remember that consistency is key to keep building momentum of your intuitive hits. I recommend regular daily practice of one or more of these exercises. These practices are super quick to do and are really helpful to build up your intuitive strength. I encourage you to set an alarm on your phone or put a Post-it note in an obvious place to help remind you to practice one or more of these exercises. Regular practice will not only strengthen your intuition, but it will also allow you to hear the intuitive guidance more easily and this will make taking action on those intuitive hits a lot easier too because you will have gradually built up more and more trust for your inner guidance.

You may find that experimenting with your own take on these exercises is very helpful too. This is a powerful way of connecting your intuition and finding out what works best for you. Developing your intuition is a personal experience so I greatly encourage you to try these exercises and to adjust and adapt them as you wish and keep experimenting to find what works for you.

It may also be helpful to keep an intuition journal. This is a notebook or even a notes app that you would use to record your experiences. Keeping notes on this can help you to see how far you've come. It will also allow you to reflect back on any insights that you have gleaned from previous exercises and even see trends for symbols that may continue to pop up over time.

Exercise 1: Direct Intuition

This exercise is similar to a meditation or breathwork practice. Head over to http://www.nourishwithrenata.com/ healyourbodymindandspirit for the follow-along video for this exercise.

Intuition speaks to you more clearly when we make space for quiet reflection time so that is what we will do now. The most important part of this exercise is to release any expectation and just allow whatever comes to your mind to come without judgment.

* Sit comfortably in a high-backed chair or cross-legged on the floor. It may be helpful to lean against a wall to help alleviate any back pain or place a pillow or cushion under your legs to help you with any potential hip pain.

* Start by rolling your shoulders a couple of times and/or rolling your neck.

* Release anything that has come before this moment and anything that is coming after this moment.

* Allow your eyelids to gently close or focus on a point that is unmoving on the floor or somewhere in front of you.

* Begin with three deep cleansing breaths.

* Deep inhale and exhale,

* Repeat two more times.

* Come back to your natural breathing pattern

* Allow your mind to quietly focus only on the inhale and the exhale.

* Now once you are relaxed and quiet, identify a situation that you would like your intuition to speak to you on. It may be helpful to ask a yes/no question to yourself like:

* "Is this the right thing to do?"

* "Should I talk to this person?"

* "Is this the right decision for me now?"

* Focus on this situation or event for a few minutes. Allow your mind's eye or any sensory feelings to happen and be the gentle observer for anything and everything that comes up.

✳ Any feelings that pop up may relate to the intuitive language that you are most accustomed to or are strengthening. Take note of the feeling. What does it feel like? What was your first instinct when this feeling came up? Was it a "no" feeling or a "yes" feeling?

✳ If nothing in particular is coming to mind, that is totally ok. Allow your mind to know that your intuition can speak to you on this in the near future as well.

✳ Once you are ready to complete the practice, set the intention to let go of your request and allow any feelings, thoughts, sensory experiences to be released from the body.

✳ Take three more cleaning breaths.

✳ Start wiggling your fingers and toes.

✳ Gently open your eyes.

Exercise 2: Indirect Intuition Exercise

This exercise contains two methods to help strengthen your indirect intuition.

Method 1: Setting a Dream Intention

This method is for right before you go to bed at night.

✳ What I'd like for you to do is take a journal and a pen or pencil and allow yourself to settle into your bed. Get cozy and comfortable.

✳ Think about a situation that you would like intuitive guidance on.

* Write down in your journal what the situation is and what you would like guidance on. Do you need guidance on what to say, what the next step is, the tone of voice you should use, how to solve a problem, etc?

* Set the intention or even say out loud or write down: I set the intention for my intuition to guide me on this situation in my dreams tonight.

* Close the journal and let it go. Allow yourself to release what you've written and what you were just thinking on and trust that your intuition will guide you in your dreams.

* When you've woken up in the morning, write down what you dreamt about. Write down the symbols and signs that you saw - don't worry about analysis right now, just write down everything that comes to mind when you reflect on your dreams.

* After you've done that brain dump of your dream, go back and look for common threads or common symbols. What sticks out to you as important? Think back to previous experiences that may have had these common threads or symbols too. What did they mean to you? Write down any and all things that come to your mind. If you don't find a common symbol or thread yet, don't worry. Something may come to mind later in the day that you can write down and reflect on too.

Remember this is a practice and it will become easier to find the symbols as you continue practicing.

Method 2: Asking for a Sign

This is a method that I first learned about from Gabby Bernstein and she used it to help get guidance from the Universe.

What I love about this method is that it allows your intuition to nudge you when this sign is around you.

✳ All you need to do is pick a sign that you would like the Universe to show you today to indicate that you are on the right path. It can be an animal, a plant, a word, pretty much anything that is of significance for you.

✳ In Gabby's book, she picked an owl. For me, I pick either a butterfly or a pink rose. These are two symbols that I love, that make me happy, and that I ask to see to remind me that I am on the right path.

✳ At the beginning of your day, or after you have been thinking about a particular situation that you have an inkling of what you might do, ask the Universe—either out loud or written down—to show you that particular symbol that you've chosen.

✳ Then let it go.

✳ Forget about it, do something else, go for a walk, have lunch, do something else and let your intuition nudge you when your sign is around.

Exercise 3: Practice your Intuitive Language

This is a great technique to strengthen the feeling of how your intuitive language speaks to you.

When those intuitive hits are clear and distinct, it becomes much easier to experience your intuition and then be able to take action based upon your intuition.

There are two methods I want to share with you: One is a stationary exercise and one is a moving exercise.

Method 1: Stationary Practice

First, choose the intuitive language that you want to work on. I recommend picking the intuitive language that resonates with you the most. For me, I tend to pick my gut feeling, or clairsentience, for this practice.

Next, ask yourself a yes/no question that you logically know the answer to. For example, is my name Renata? Feel into how your intuition responds during the split second after you ask the question. The answer to my question is clearly a yes, so for me in my gut, it feels like it is a lifting feeling from my belly button area towards my chest, right under my rib cage. What does a yes feel like for you?

It may be helpful to write down what the feeling is, or put it into words in an effort to almost explain it to yourself.

You can also repeat asking a question to yourself where the answer is no, for instance, am I a dog? Pay attention to how your intuition responds immediately following this No question. For me it feels like a sinking or dropping feeling, from my belly button area, down to the pelvic floor. It's not a draining feeling, based upon the question being quite superficial, but it is a distinct dropping or lowering feeling.

What does your no feeling feel like? Once again, write it down or try to explain it in words to yourself. This really does help you create stronger connections with how your intuition feels in your body.

Method 2: Moving Exercise

This is a method I like to use when going for a walk alone in nature or around my neighborhood.

When you get to an intersection, ask your intuition which way you should go. Listen for that quick split-second answer on which direction you should turn.

I often feel a lightness or a lifting in my belly telling me to turn left vs right or I will feel a pull to turn right vs left. It really is as simple as that. Of course, don't let yourself go into any unsafe areas of town, but allow your intuition to make choices on what path to walk today. And as always, your intuition may speak to you differently, depending on the exercise that you choose to do today to strengthen it or it may start a new intuitive language speaking to you.

When practicing strengthening your intuition, remember to take action based upon what your intuition is telling you. For me, this is the way to close the loop, so to speak, when it comes to your intuition. The whole point of your intuition is to let it guide you in your life, so if you don't take action on what your intuition is telling you, what's the point? Take action on what your intuition is telling you and watch the strength of your intuition grow!

We are Energy

We are energetic beings. Every single cell in our body is made up of atoms, or little tiny vibrating particles that are pure energy. Light is energy waves and colors are made up of different frequencies of light energy waves. Sounds are energy waves with different pitches of sound at different frequencies of sound waves. Even thoughts in our brains are electronic signals between cells that have been measured through electroencephalography (EEG). Everything we are and everything that we do is made up of energy. But more than that, what we put into our body, like food, drink, the media we watch, and podcasts we listen to are all made up of energy. So, we are literally feeding ourselves energy all day, every day in some form or another.

The question is, are you aware of the energy that you are putting into your body? And are you aware of the impact that this energy can have on you?

The energy that we allow to affect us, consciously or subconsciously, can influence how we feel, think, and act. Have you ever talked to someone and felt like they really drained your energy just by speaking to them? Or perhaps you've walked into a room of people and instantly felt so much happier and joyful without understanding why? These are all great examples of how the energy in a room or the energy of people can really affect our own energy.

Most people go through life thinking that they cannot control how other's energy affects them. But that is actually not the case. You can become more aware of other's energy and make a decision on how much you let it affect you. You can also learn how the energy of food and drink affects your body. This knowledge allows you to have a more mindful approach to how you respond versus react to the situations that occur around you daily and how you allow, or don't allow, these situations to affect your choices for nourishment. This gives you an opportunity to shift and change your current reality to support you in your lifelong journey to healing your body, mind, and spirit.

What are Chakras and are they Real?

I was introduced to the idea of chakras many years ago but was not convinced that they were real, so I set out to do some research to figure out if what people were saying were true.

The chakras are a system that first originated in India between 1500 to 500 BC in the Vedas, an ancient sacred text of spiritual knowledge. It was passed down verbally to new generations until New Age authors expanded on these old texts and made the chakra system more widely known.

The Sanskrit word chakra means wheel. A chakra is often thought of as a rotating wheel of energy and can sometimes be denoted as a lotus flower. Each chakra is believed to vibrate at its own frequency in a circular pattern. These frequencies of vibration can be altered to help keep the body in homeostasis. The chakras are related to the energetic body with some relation of the main seven chakras to certain physical body organs. The psychologist Richard Maxwell proposed that chakras are the channels between cytoplasm of two adjacent cells that allow for communication and passage of ions, molecules, and electrical impulses. Specifically, chakras tend to align with regions of the body with higher density of intracellular gap junctions that were created during development of the embryo. Maxwell's theory expands upon the scientific work of Charles Shang that explained that chakras and meridians come from intracellular networks between undifferentiated cells involved in embryological development.

There are seven main chakras that run along the spine, and some people believe up to 114 chakras throughout the whole body. It is believed that the health of a chakra is directly connected to physical, mental, and emotional health as well. It seems that originally, chakras were a meditative aid, particularly part of a meditative exercise that became yoga. As yoga became more popular in Western culture, so did the chakra system, and it seemed to start to attract more interpretation and supplementary tools such as essential oils, crystals, and specific colors for each chakra.

The main seven energy centers or chakras are the Crown, Third Eye, Throat, Heart, Solar Plexus, Sacral and Root Chakras.

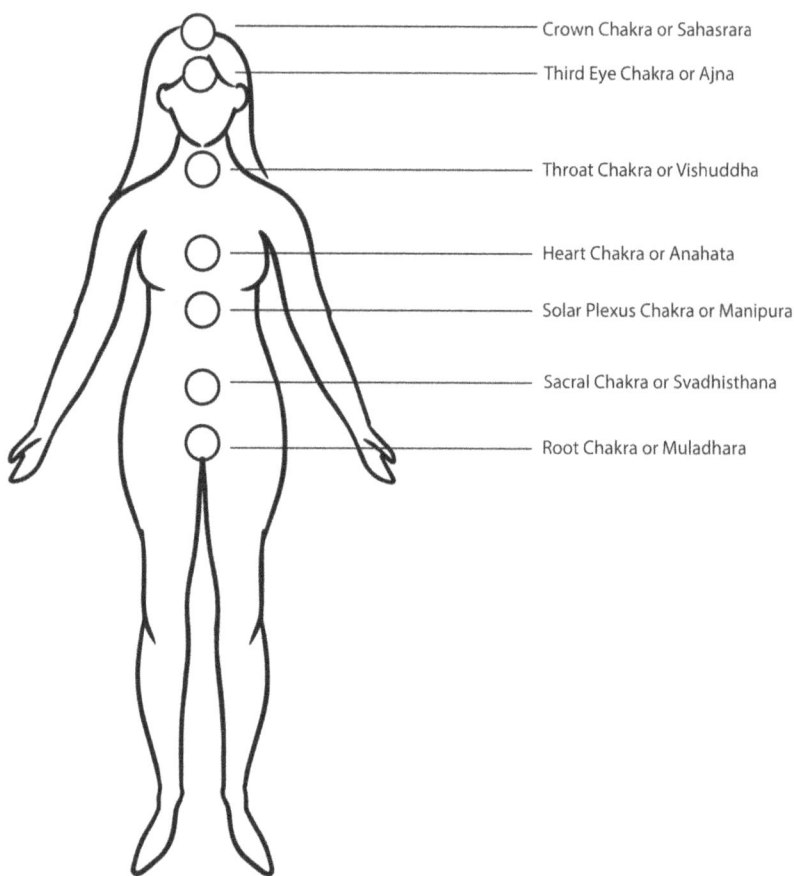

Crown Chakra or Sahasrara

Third Eye Chakra or Ajna

Throat Chakra or Vishuddha

Heart Chakra or Anahata

Solar Plexus Chakra or Manipura

Sacral Chakra or Svadhisthana

Root Chakra or Muladhara

Scientific studies into the functional theories of chakras indicate that chakras are linked to the central nervous system. For instance, the crown chakra is linked with the neocortex, the third eye with the prefrontal cortex, the throat chakra with the limbic system, the heart chakra with the midbrain, the solar plexus with the pons, and the sacral and root chakras with the medulla oblongata. These chakras provide the mind with brain-body structures that indicate the status of the central nervous system.

The science behind chakras is still emerging and more research will likely be needed to further explain some of the qualitative experiences that people experience. The first item to note is, as mentioned previously, our whole body is made up of energy, specifically electrical energy. Our nervous system and brains are electro-chemical machines. Our bodies are also made up of approximately 70% water, which is a great electric conductor. Blood is an even better electrical conductor which is why every heartbeat creates an electrical pulse throughout the whole circulatory system which is measured by an electrocardiogram or ECG.

Electrical conduction involves the transfer of electrons which can occur through strong magnetism. When electricity and magnetism interact, an electromagnetic field in and around the body is measurable. Every organ, in fact every human cell, has its own electromagnetic field. These electromagnetic fields form a whole electromagnetic field around the whole human being.

This electromagnetic field is also called a biofield by the National Institute of Health, NIH. It is the field of energy and information that surrounds and interpenetrates the human body.

This electromagnetic field, whether around the whole human or around specific organs, may not be able to be seen by the human eye or other human senses, so this makes it challenging to use science to quantitatively measure, but there continues to be research into this to further explain the impact of these electromagnetic fields on our overall wellbeing. For instance, quantum physics has been looking at cells and body systems and seeing that they are actually constantly in motion, trying to find homeostasis. Our cells are constantly vibrating, even though we cannot physically see this with our eye or acknowledge this with our other human senses. Despite not being able to physically acknowledge this vibration, science has been able to show us that this is indeed happening. If this is happening, who is to say that the chakras, or energetic wheels rotating with its own vibration, are not also a part of our energetic bodies?

I believe that this is just one example that the level of our science is slowly expanding to be able to prove some things that Eastern beliefs have been teaching for centuries. This is why we are seeing more of an integrative or holistic approach to medicine in recent years aka an understanding that we need both a scientific approach to medicine as well as a holistic and spiritual approach in order to fully examine, analyze and possibly even prevent illness in the physical body from occurring. This methodology is called integrative medicine with a particular branch being energy medicine, which aims to understand the energetic body through therapeutic techniques. Continuing research[15] in energy medicine will look at the overlap of the endocrine and chakra systems and dive deeper into how energy medicine enhances psychoneuroimmunology medicine aka the mind-body immune response.

The 7 Main Chakras

Now for a deep dive into the seven main chakras and the importance of each plus the organs they may relate to in the physical body.

The Root Chakra or Muladhara in Sanskrit

This chakra is commonly called the first chakra. It is located at the base of your spine. The Root Chakra supports your foundation for life, stability, security and your resilience to challenges. It is related to your physical identity and your sense of sure-footedness. Often associated with Grounding and your connection with the Earth.

The Root Chakra is typically associated with the color red.

The Sacral Chakra or Svadhisthana

This chakra is located around the sexual organs, such as the womb space in women and the penis and testes in men. This chakra is not only related to sensuality and sexuality—it is also the center for creative energy. It is the emotional center for yourself and how you relate to others.

The Sacral Chakra is associated with an orange color.

The Solar Plexus or Manipura

This chakra is located around your stomach area and is your powerhouse center. It is where you get all your internal power, confidence, and self-esteem from.

The Solar Plexus Chakra is associated with the color yellow, distinct, vibrant, and bold.

The Heart Chakra or Anahata

Located around your heart space, this chakra is often referred to as the Heart Center. This chakra is all about love in relationships with others and self, as well as compassion.

The Heart Chakra is associated with the color green. It is also the middle of the main seven chakras so it connects what is referred to as the lower chakras (Root, Sacral and Solar Plexus) and the upper chakras (Throat, Third Eye and Crown).

The Throat Chakra or Vishudda

The Throat Chakra is located in your throat where your vocal cords are. It relates to your communication and speaking your truth. It is all about clarity as well as self-expression with ease and grace.

The Throat Chakra is associated with the color blue.

The Third Eye Chakra or Ajna

This chakra is located between the eyebrows and an inch or two behind the skin of the forehead. The Third Eye Chakra relates to intuition, imagination and visualization. This chakra helps us to envision ideas prior to creating them in the physical world.

It is commonly associated with an Indigo color.

The Crown Chakra or Sahasrara

The Crown Chakra is located at the top of your head. It is related to your spiritual connection. This could be to a power greater than yourself and your connection to yourself and others. It is also connected to all the other chakras.

This chakra is often associated with a violet or a white color.

Chakra Balance

In daily life, it is easy for our chakras to get out of balance. Influence from the world around us or from other people, can have a range of impact on your body and thus, your energy centers. When our chakras are out of balance for too long, this may manifest itself in physical ailments and disease. It can also affect your emotional health and wellbeing.

Here is a brief synopsis of some symptoms you may experience if your chakras are out of balance:

Root Chakra Imbalance

✳ Digestive issues such as constipation, excessive bowel movements, colon problems, bladder issues, etc

✳ Arthritis

✳ Feeling fearful, worried and insecure about your basic needs such as shelter, security, food, money, etc

✳ Feeling aggressive, greed, or attachment to things, people, or outcomes

Sacral Chakra Imbalance

✳ Pelvic pain/issues

✳ Urinary tract infections

✳ Lower back pain

✳ Impotency

✳ Low feelings of self-worth

✳ Not feeling pleasure or sensualness

✳ Lack of creativity

✳ Codependence

Solar Plexus Chakra Imbalance

* Indigestion

* Stomach pain and discomfort

* Heartburn

* Stomach ulcers

* Low self-esteem and self-confidence

* Lack of belief in self and your own power

* Lack of decision making

* Acting obsessively or having an unhealthy need to control

Heart Chakra Imbalance

* Heart problems (physical and emotional) such as heart attacks or the feeling of a broken heart after a relationship ending

* Asthma or other breathing problems

* Weight gain due to poor relationship with self and food.

* Feelings of loneliness, insecurity and isolation

* Feelings of defensiveness, jealousy, holding grudges, guilt, and shame

Throat Chakra Imbalance

* Vocal issues such as hoarseness, losing your voice, etc

* Cough or other throat problems e.g. laryngitis, thyroid issues, temporomandibular joint (TMJ), tickle in your throat that you cannot get rid of, etc

* Mouth issues such as teeth, gum disease, ulcers, or other dental issues.

* Having trouble speaking your mind or on the flip side, dominating conversations, lying, or gossiping

Third Eye Chakra Imbalance

* Headaches and migraines

* Issues with sight

* Concentration problems

* Hearing issues: physical as well as selective hearing

* Not sensing your intuition or how it speaks to you

* Feeling stuck in your life, career, relationships, etc

* Lack of clarity or vision in your life, career, relationships, etc

Crown Chakra

* Narrow mindedness, skepticism and stubbornness

* Disconnection from a spiritual practice

* Apathy

* Materialism

How to Re-balance Your Chakras

For optimal health, physically, emotionally and spiritually, your chakras need to be aligned. You can do this on a daily basis or as frequently as you need during the course of one day.

There are several different methods that can help you to align your chakras. Some of them are:

* Meditation

* Breathwork

* Journaling

* Essential oils

* Certain yoga postures can target a particular chakra or even doing your favorite yoga flow may be helpful

* Prayer

* Tibetan bowls or similar sound healing

* Speaking to a trusted friend or family member or a professional

* Any movement that is soothing and helpful to release tension and anything that is on your mind in a mindful way e.g. walking in nature, tai chi, qi gong, etc

All of these methods are helpful for you to release any stress and tension that you may be holding on to. When you release these emotions and physical tension, it allows your energy to travel more easily throughout your physical body and all of your energetic centers or chakras. When your energy does not flow easily through your energetic and physical bodies, it is often referred to as the energy getting "stuck" or stagnant in one area. This can lead to a chakra imbalance or out of alignment.

My favorite way of aligning my chakras was taught to me by a couple of my coaches and this simple meditation technique, which I will describe below, is a combination of the techniques. It should take you about ten minutes, depending on how mindfully you connect with each of your chakras. You can also listen and watch the video of this meditation at http://www.nourishwithrenata.com/healyourbodymindandspirit

If you've never meditated or done a visualization before, let me explain the power behind visualization. Some of the professions we look up to the most actually use visualization. Think about athletes like Olympic level track stars, football players, and golfers use visualization to imagine their bodies performing the feats that they wish to in order to win the race, make the touchdown or hit a hole-in-one. The practice of doing these visualizations over and over again actually impacts the brain since the brain cannot tell the difference between what is a lived experience vs what is an imagined experience. As a result, the Reticular Activating System, RAS, in the brain marks this repeated thought as important, and then goes about finding evidence in daily life to confirm that this visualized result can be true in our current reality. It causes our decision-making processes to change and adapt in order to ensure the visualized outcome. Visualizing is an important tool of the subconscious mind to embed desires into our brains so that our current reality changes and becomes what we want.

Practicing visualization, or guided meditation, is the repetition of a thought or series of thoughts that indicates to the brain that this is important and the end result we desire needs to be brought into the current reality. This practice of clearing the chakras, or releasing any pent-up negative energy, tells our brains it is important to release stress and tension so that I can feel more aligned and peaceful as a result.

I highly encourage you to try visualization or guided meditations and observe how you feel afterwards. Be open to trying it if you've never done it before and be aware of how this impacts your energy, reactiveness, and the rest of your day.

Meditation to Clear Your Energy and Balance Your Chakras

To follow along with me as I guide this meditation, go to http:// www.nourishwithrenata.com/healyourbodymindandspirit

First, start off in a comfortable cross-legged position or sitting in a chair with a straight back. If you are sitting in a chair, allow your feet to rest flat on the floor. Turn your palms so that they face upwards; this is a physical position that allows the body to be open to receive.

Gently allow your eyes to close as you take in three deep breaths, all the way down in the belly button. Exhale fully through the mouth, allowing the belly button to pull all the way towards the spine so that the breath fully escapes. Repeat this three times.

Keeping your eyes closed, imagine that about eighteen inches above your head, there is a bright white orb of light floating. This is called your Soul Star. It is your connection to God, the Universe, or any higher power that you believe in.

Imagine there is a cord of light emanating down from the Soul Star that travels down and connects with the very top of your head, right at your Crown Chakra. As the light touches your Crown Chakra, the Crown Chakra is lit up with the same bright white light that clears any negative energy, stress, or tension from this chakra. Imagine that the chakra is rotating in a clockwise direction and spins faster as the negative energy is cleared. If you feel any tension in the area where your chakra is located, then allow the chakra to increase in size slightly until you feel the chakra is no longer dampened. Imagine the color of the light intensifies as it clears, heals, balances, and aligns this chakra.

If a chakra feels very open and expansive, this can be a sign to start reducing the size of the chakra and slowing down the rotation of the chakra. This is something that can help you to protect your energy more, especially if there is an energetic leak happening through this chakra.

Allow the bright white light of the Soul Star to move its way down to your Third Eye Chakra, between your eyebrows, and a little further back into the head towards your pituitary gland, located at the center of the lowermost side of the brain. You may imagine a violet disc of light at this point, gently rotating in the clockwise direction, and potentially increasing in size if you wish to open up this chakra more.

Bring the bright white light down past the eyes, nose, ears, and mouth, lighting up those areas along the way to the Throat Chakra. This Chakra is all about communication of self. With this chakra, imagine a blue disc of light rotating in a clockwise fashion, clearing, aligning and healing energetic blocks or releasing any negative energy. Increase or decrease the speed of rotation, and/or the size of the chakra based upon how you feel this chakra is. You may feel a tightness in your throat if you are finding it challenging to express yourself fully. That then will be released as you mindfully visualize this chakra gently opening.

The bright white light of the Soul Star begins to travel down the shoulders, releasing the tension held in this area, then moves into the heart space or the Heart Chakra. The chakra in this area is lit up with a green light that rotates in a clockwise direction and can be opened/closed, or the speed of rotation can change, depending on how you are feeling. Ensure that any tension, stress, overwhelm, frustration, etc is being released as the bright, white light moves into the chakra. Set the intention to heal, balance, and align this chakra using the Soul Star light.

The light moves down to your stomach area, just below the rib cage, where your Solar Plexus Chakra is located. This is your Powerhouse Chakra, which is colored with bright yellow. Heal, balance, and align this chakra, increasing or decreasing the rate of rotation of the chakra, intensifying the light as you see fit in order to release any negative energy, stress or tension that may be held here. We often hold in our stomachs during the day anyway, so this is a great opportunity to breathe and relax—to let go. As your chakra is cleared and strengthened using the bright, white light of the Soul Star, this will in turn help you to increase your feelings of self-worth and confidence—your power is literally being restored.

Bring the Soul Star light down into your Sacral Chakra, also known as roughly where the sexual organs are e.g. the uterus for women, and the penis and testes for men. This chakra is your creativity house. Allow the light to clear, balance, and align your chakra, adjusting the speed and size of the chakra to ensure that the chakra is healed, balanced, and aligned. Feel your creativity rise as the orange color of this chakra returns.

Now the bright, white light of the Soul Star moves down to the base of the spine where your Root Chakra is located. This chakra is all about stability and security. It is your foundation. Allow the light to cleanse the chakra, releasing stress, worry, frustration, doubt. Set the intention to heal balance and align this chakra. Feel the muscles in the body in this area relax and soften. Feel the base of the spine become grounded and melt into the Earth or the chair that you are sitting on.

Once these seven chakras have had the Soul Star light move through them, allow the light to run down the legs, and into the Earth. Imagine that the light moves down through all the different layers of the Earth and towards the very core of the Earth.

At the core of the Earth, the light meets with the energy of Mother Earth, a deeply held, loving, grounding energy that infuses itself into the light from the Soul Star. This combined energy and light moves back up the different layers of the Earth and back up to your feet.

This renewed and reinvigorated light and energy moves back up through your legs and into your Root Chakra, infusing it with this new light and energy. Bring the light up to the Sacral Chakra to enlighten it, then to the Solar Plexus Chakra where the light reinvigorates your core. The light moves up to the Heart Chakra, lighting it up with this new energy, and then to the Throat Chakra, lighting up your throat space. Move this light up to the Third Eye Chakra, igniting the forehead once more before finally back up to the Crown Chakra, where you visualize seeing the top of the head lit up with this beautiful Mother Earth energy. Finally, bring the light back up to the Soul Star. You are connected above as you are below. Your body is free and released of the previous energies that were draining you. You are completely relaxed, lit up with new light and energy, and ready to make today incredible.

To end the meditation, take three more deep breaths down to the belly button. Inhaling through the nose, fill up the lungs, and allow the belly to expand as it fills up also. Hold for a second, then exhale through the mouth, making a big sigh or noise as you do so. Repeat this two more times and on the last breath in, hold that inhale for as long as possible. Then exhale fully and completely, pulling the belly button to the spine to ensure all the breath has escaped. Resume your natural breathing pattern. Start to wiggle your fingers and toes, and, when you're ready, gently flutter your eyelids open.

You are ready to take on the rest of your day.

Food for your Chakras

Food is a powerful way of helping you to support and balance your chakras. As we have already discussed, food is a powerful healing tool, and can be even more useful when it comes to aligning your chakras. This is truly a wonderful way to bring together the physical, energetic, and spiritual bodies for the ultimate body, mind, and spirit healing.

In the following pages, I have included ingredients and recipes that can support each of the main seven chakras. After doing the guided meditation above, or if you're noticing any areas of the body that are experiencing some discomfort, or need extra support for the related chakra, refer to these recipes and ingredients. They are easy to add to your day to allow you to have a holistic way to support your health, body, and energy.

The Root Chakra

To help support the Root Chakra, lean into foods that are the color red. Fruits and vegetables such as red apples, tomatoes, red berries like strawberries and raspberries, radishes, and pomegranates are all great options.

In addition, root vegetables are a literal translation of the Root Chakra to help with additional grounding. Root vegetables are ingredients such as sweet potatoes, turnips, carrots, beets, and parsnips, as well as root spices such as ginger and turmeric. Root vegetables are typically high in many vitamins and minerals, such as antioxidants, Vitamin C, beta-carotene, and fiber, and are a slower release carbohydrate source. Root spices, such as turmeric, have been shown to be an incredibly powerful anti-inflammatory spice, as well as anti-cancer and anti-fungal[16]. Pair it with a healthy fat and a pinch of black pepper to increase your absorption of the active compound in turmeric, curcumin, up to 2000%. Ginger is also a flavorful addition to meals and has been helpful with calming stomach upset. Other naturally-colored red spices are also great for this chakra, such as paprika and cayenne pepper.

Protein has grounding properties, perfect for supporting the Root Chakra. Incorporating different varieties of protein, such as both animal-sourced and plant-based, can be helpful for getting a wider range of amino acids in your eating plan, depending on your eating preference. Examples of animal-sourced proteins are red meat, chicken, turkey, fish, and shellfish. Plant-based protein sources are beans, legumes, nuts, and seeds.

ROOT CHAKRA RECIPES

Roasted Beet Salad
with Raspberry Vinaigrette

Servings: 2 people

Ingredients

1–2lbs of beets
1 Tbsp avocado oil
1 tsp salt
4 cups arugula
½ red onion, finely sliced

For the Raspberry Vinaigrette

¼ cup fresh raspberries
Up to 1 Tbsp stevia or monk fruit sweetener.
1 lemon, halved
1 tsp salt
½ tsp black pepper
¼ cup extra virgin olive oil

Instructions

1.   Preheat the oven to 375°F.

2.   Wash and gently scrub the outside of the beets to remove any dirt. We will not be removing the skins of the beets since they are edible and are a great source of fiber.

3.   Dry the beets.

4.   Slice the beets into eighths (as in eight wedges for each beet).

5. On a large rimmed baking sheet, place the beets and drizzle over the avocado oil and salt. Gently toss together to combine well.

6. Roast in the preheated oven for about 35–45 mins or until the beets are tender and have a deep red hue.

7. Meanwhile, to make the raspberry vinaigrette, add the raspberries, monk fruit sweetener, juice from the lemon, salt, pepper, and olive oil into a blender or food processor.

8. Blend well until smooth.

9. Taste and adjust seasonings as desired. Depending on the sweetness of the raspberries, you may want to add more stevia or monk fruit sweetener to balance the potential tartness of the raspberries.

10. To assemble the salad, divide the arugula on two plates, top with beets, a scattering of red onion slices, and drizzle the raspberry vinaigrette over it.

Golden Vegetable Soup with Crispy Chickpeas

Servings: 4 people

Ingredients

For the Golden Turmeric Vegetable Soup

1 Tbsp olive oil
1 large onion, finely diced
1 large carrot, diced
2 stalks celery, diced
3 cloves garlic, minced
½ Tbsp ground turmeric
1 tsp ground cumin
½ tsp ground coriander
14 oz green lentils rinsed, drained and any bits removed
5 cups low-sodium vegetable broth
1 (13.5 oz) can coconut milk, shaken well
Salt and pepper to taste
1 cup chopped kale, optional

For the Crispy Chickpeas

1 can of chickpeas, drained, rinsed and dried
   on kitchen towels
1 Tbsp olive oil
1 tsp salt
½ tsp black pepper

Instructions

For the Golden Turmeric Vegetable Soup

1. In a large saucepan, heat olive oil over medium-high heat.
2. Add onions and sauté until tender and starting to turn golden brown.
3. Add carrots and celery and stir.
4. Add in garlic and stir until fragrant, about 1 minute.
5. Now add in the turmeric, cumin, and coriander.
6. Add in the lentils and stir until well combined.
7. Slowly pour in the broth and stir thoroughly.
8. Lower the heat to medium low and allow the soup to simmer until the lentils are softened, about 15 minutes.
9. Pour in the coconut milk and stir until well combined. Add in kale, if desired.
10. Taste the soup and add salt and pepper to taste.
11. If desired, garnish with Crispy Chickpeas before serving.

For the Crispy Chickpeas

1. Preheat the oven to 400°F.
2. On a large rimmed baking sheet, add the dried chickpeas.
3. Drizzle the olive oil, salt, and pepper, and toss to combine.
4. Roast in the preheated oven for about 40 minutes, tossing the chickpeas halfway through the cooking time.
5. Roast the chickpeas until they are crispy and golden brown.
6. Remove from the oven and use them to top the Golden Turmeric Vegetable Soup.

Citrus-Marinated Chicken
with Roasted Red Pepper Hummus

Servings: 4 people

Ingredients

4 chicken breasts, halved horizontally to reduce the
    thickness of the chicken breast

1 orange

1 lemon

1 lime

2 cloves of garlic, smashed and skin removed

2 tsp salt

1 tsp black pepper

2 Tbsp + 1 tsp avocado oil

8 cups of your favorite salad greens, such as baby kale,
    spinach, frisee, etc

For the Roasted Red Pepper Hummus

1 can chickpeas, drained and rinsed

½ cup roasted red peppers, drained of any liquid in the jar

1 garlic clove, peeled

¼ cup tahini

1 tsp salt

½ tsp black pepper

¼–½ cup of extra virgin olive oil

Instructions

1. In a large container or resealable bag, place the chicken
   breasts. Add the zest and juice of the orange, lemon and
   lime, plus the garlic, salt, pepper and avocado oil.

2. Seal the container or resealable bag and place in the
   refrigerator for at least 1 hour and up to 24 hours before
   cooking. The longer the chicken is left in the marinade,
   the more tender and flavorful it will be.

3. When ready to cook, preheat a large sauté pan over medium heat. Add 1 tsp avocado oil.

4. Remove the chicken breast from the marinade, allowing any excess marinade to drip off.

5. Carefully place the chicken breast into the preheated sauté pan.

6. Repeat the last two steps with as many chicken breast pieces as will fit in the pan in one layer.

7. Cook until the chicken breast is golden brown on the underside, approximately 4-5 minutes depending on the thickness of the slices.

8. Carefully flip over the chicken breast pieces and repeat on the second side. Cook until golden brown on the underside and the chicken is cooked through or the internal temperature is 165°F.

9. Meanwhile, for the Roasted Red Pepper Hummus, place the chickpeas, roasted red peppers, garlic, tahini, salt, and pepper into a food processor or blender. Blend until the mixture is coming together. It could be quite thick at this stage and may require you to use a spatula to scrape the sides of the blender or food processor bowl to reincorporate any ingredients.

10. While the blender is running, slowly pour in the olive oil to create a creamy texture.

11. Taste and adjust seasonings if desired.

12. To serve, per person, place about 2 cups of the salad greens on a plate. Top with one of the cooked chicken breasts and then add a spoonful of the roasted red pepper hummus. Enjoy warm!

Strawberry Rosewater Protein Smoothie

Servings: 1 person

Ingredients

1 Tbsp chia seeds
1 Tbsp flax seeds
⅓ cup fresh or frozen strawberries
1 tsp rose water
½ cup riced cauliflower, frozen
1 scoop vanilla protein powder
1 cup of ice
1–2 cups milk of your choice

Instructions

1. Add all the ingredients in a high-speed blender. For a thicker smoothie, you may want to add 1 cup of your milk of choice, or if you'd like a thinner consistency add up to 2 cups of milk. You may also want to reduce the amount of ice if using both frozen strawberries and cauliflower.

2. Place the lid on the blender and carefully blend the ingredients until very smooth.

3. Enjoy immediately!

Creamy Berry Nice Cream

Ingredients

1 banana, sliced into pieces and frozen
1 cup frozen berries of choice e.g., strawberries, raspberries, blueberries, or a mixture of these

Instructions

1. To a blender, add the banana and frozen berries of choice.

2. Place the lid on the blender. If you have a tamper device, you will want to insert this into the lid of the blender, or be ready to scrape the inside of the blender several times during the next phase.

3. Carefully blend the banana and berries, using the tamper to push the frozen ingredients towards the blade, or stopping the blender and using a spatula to scrape the insides of the blender to reincorporate the ingredients. Continue doing so until a creamy ice cream texture is achieved.

4. Serve immediately!

Visit
http://www.
nourishwithrenata.com/
healyourbodymind
andspirit
for exclusive bonuses
and videos.

The Sacral Chakra

Orange-colored foods are fantastic for supporting this chakra. Vegetables like butternut squash, orange bell peppers, sweet potatoes, and carrots, plus fruits like oranges, mango, peaches and apricots, are great options. The beta-carotene, a powerful antioxidant in both fruits and vegetables, helps the body by reducing free radicals which can damage our cells. Beta-carotene has also been linked with improved eye health.

Omega-3s, the anti-inflammatory essential fatty acid, is also helpful for this chakra. Foods like wild-caught fatty fish are great for Omega-3s. Salmon, halibut, tuna, mackerel, etc are perfect for this, in addition to nuts and seeds like flax seeds, chia seeds, almonds, and walnuts. Omega-3s also help improve cardiovascular health.

Cinnamon is a fantastic spice for not only helping to balance blood sugar levels and its delicious sweet aroma and flavor but an additional support for the sacral chakra.

Good quality dark chocolate, preferably made with honey or another sugar substitute as opposed to traditional sugar, is not only pleasurable to eat, but great for the sacral chakra support too. Dark chocolate, rich in antioxidants and flavonoids, has been shown in numerous scientific studies to help relieve stress and lower inflammation.

The sacral chakra is also supported with lots of hydration. Drinking plenty of water, and having hydrating foods, such as high-water content fruits and vegetables (watermelon, strawberries, oranges, tomatoes, cucumber, celery etc) plus soups, broths and stews, are really helpful for maintaining hydration no matter the season.

Watermelon Lime Collagen Slushies

Servings: 2 people

Instructions

4 cups of fresh or frozen watermelon

1 cup water (if using frozen watermelon)

1 large lime, zested and juiced

2 servings collagen powder

2 cups ice, if not using frozen watermelon

1–2 Tbsp stevia or monk fruit sweetener, depending on the sweetness of your watermelon

Instructions

1. Place all ingredients, except stevia or monk fruit sweetener, into a high-speed blender.

2. Blend until a slushy-like consistency is achieved.

3. Taste and see if you need to add any sweetener. If so, add the sweetener and blend again.

4. Pour into glasses and enjoy immediately.

Roasted Sweet Potatoes with Kale and Horseradish Chimichurri

Servings: 4 people

Ingredients

3–4 large sweet potatoes, washed thoroughly and dried

2 tbsp avocado oil

2 tsp salt

1 tsp black pepper

For the Kale and Horseradish Chimichurri

½ cup kale, very finely chopped

2 tsp–1 Tbsp horseradish, depending on spice level desired

½ cup extra virgin olive oil

2 tbsp lemon juice

3 cloves garlic, finely minced

1 tbsp chopped fresh chilies

¾ tsp dried oregano

1 tsp salt

½ tsp black pepper

Instructions

1. Preheat the oven to 425°F.

2. Cut the washed and dried sweet potatoes into 8 wedges each.

3. Place the sweet potato wedges on a large rimmed baking sheet. You may need two baking sheets to distribute the wedges in one even layer on each tray.

4. Drizzle over the avocado oil, salt, and pepper. Toss thoroughly to coat each of the wedges.

5. Roast the sweet potato wedges in the preheated oven until crisp around the edges and tender, about 20–30 minutes.

6. Meanwhile, in a medium-sized bowl, add all the ingredients, starting with 2 tsp of horseradish, and mix well.

7. Taste and add more horseradish as desired.

8. To serve, place the sweet potato wedges on a plate and transfer some of the Kale and Horseradish Chimichurri into a small bowl to place alongside the wedges.

9. Keep any leftovers in an airtight container in the fridge for up to 1 week.

Butternut Squash Soup with Cinnamon and Vanilla

Servings: 4 people

Ingredients

1 large butternut squash
1 Tbsp olive oil
1 onion, diced
2 stalks of celery, diced
2 cloves of garlic, minced
8 cups of vegetable broth
2 tsp salt
1 tsp black pepper
½ tsp cinnamon
1 tsp vanilla extract

Instructions

1. Carefully cut the top and bottom portion of the butternut squash off. This will create a level surface on the bottom which will make the butternut squash easier to peel and dice.

2. Cut the less bulbous, stem portion of the butternut squash off.

3. Using your knife, carefully cut off the skin on the stem portion of the butternut squash.

4. Once the skin has been removed, chop the butternut squash into roughly 2" chunks.

5. Repeat the last two steps with the bulbous section of the butternut squash, taking a few extra minutes to remove the butternut squash seeds too.

6. Preheat a large Dutch oven, or a large pot with a lid, over medium heat.

7. Add the olive oil.

8. Once hot, add the onion and celery, and sauté until softened, about 5 mins.

9. Add the garlic and stir until fragrant, about 1 minute.

10. Add the chopped butternut squash, then pour over the vegetable broth.

11. Bring the soup to a boil, reduce the heat to a simmer, then place the lid on the pot.

12. Simmer until the butternut squash is tender, about 20–25 mins depending on the size of the butternut squash that you've cut.

13. Now it is time to blend the soup to create a creamy texture. There are two methods:

    a. **Immersion blender method:** Using an immersion blender, carefully blend the soup in the pot (heat should be turned off) until the soup is creamy and thick.

    b. **Blender method:** Take portions of the soup and put into a high-speed blender. Remove the insert from the lid of the blender then place the lid on the blender. Cover the opening in the lid with a folded kitchen towel to protect yourself from being splashed with hot soup as it blends. Ensure the lid is tightly on the blender and keep your hand on the lid as you carefully start the blender. Blend until the soup is smooth and creamy. Pour the blended portion of the soup in a large container, then blend the remaining soup in the same manner until all the soup has been blended. Pour all the soup back in the pot.

14. Add in the cinnamon and vanilla extract to the soup. Stir well.

15. Taste and add additional seasonings if desired.

16. Serve warm.

Honey Chipotle Salmon with Lemon Dijon Rice Salad

Servings: 4 people

For the Lemon Dijon Salad

2 cups leftover cold rice (carefully break apart any large clumps of cold rice)
2 cups sugar snap peas, chopped
1 Tbsp olive oil
2 red or yellow bell peppers, cut into 1/2-inch-thick strips
2 zucchinis, chopped into large chunks
1 tsp salt
½ tsp black pepper

For the Lemon Dijon Dressing

1 large lemon, juiced and zested
¼ cup extra virgin olive oil
1 tsp Dijon mustard
1 tsp salt
½ tsp black pepper

For the Honey Chipotle Salmon

4 filets of salmon
1 Tbsp honey
¼ tsp chipotle chili powder (or use regular chili powder)
1 Tbsp avocado oil
Salt and freshly ground black pepper to taste

Instructions

For the Lemon Dijon Rice Salad

1. Preheat the oven to 400°F.

2. Take a large rimmed baking tray and place the chopped bell peppers and zucchini on it.

3. Drizzle over olive oil, salt and pepper and toss to combine.

4. Roast for approx. 30 minutes until the vegetables are tender and caramelized along the edges.

5. Remove from the oven and allow to cool.

6. Meanwhile, add the ingredients for the Lemon Dijon Dressing in a jar with a tight-fitting lid.

7. Tighten the lid and shake the jar vigorously to combine.

8. Once the roasted vegetables have cooled, add the cooled rice, roasted vegetables, chopped sugar snap peas, and the dressing to a large bowl. Toss thoroughly to combine.

For the Honey Chipotle Salmon

1. In a small bowl, whisk together the honey, chipotle powder, oil, salt, and pepper. Set aside.

2. Heat a large sauté pan over medium high heat.

3. Once the pan is hot, add the salmon, flesh side down, and cook for approximately 4-5 minutes or until the underside is golden brown and a crust has developed.

4. Carefully turn the salmon over and cook until the desired doneness.

5. Meanwhile, glaze the top side of the salmon with the honey-chipotle mixture.

6. Once the salmon is cooked to your liking, remove the salmon from the pan and glaze once more with the honey-chipotle mixture.

7. To serve, add some of the Lemon Dijon Rice salad to a plate and top with a salmon filet. Enjoy!

Sacral Breakfast Cookies

Servings: 12 cookies

Ingredients

2 Tbsp chia seeds

5 Tbsp water

2 cups gluten free oats

2 Tbsp monk fruit sweetener

1 cup grated carrots

1 banana, mashed

1 tsp vanilla extract

½ cup tahini (sesame seed paste)

¹/₃ cup stevia sweetened chocolate chips

Zest and Juice of 1 mandarin orange

1 tsp ground cinnamon

Instructions

1. Preheat the oven to 350°F.

2. In a small bowl, add the chia seeds and water. Stir and then allow to sit for 5 minutes to thicken.

3. In a large bowl, add the oats, monk fruit sweetener, carrots, banana, vanilla extract, and tahini. Mix well to combine.

4. Add the chia seed-water mixture to the large bowl and then stir again to thoroughly combine.

5. Finally add the chocolate chips and mix into the batter.

6. Take 2 cookie sheets and line with parchment paper or a non-stick mat.

7. Scoop tablespoons of the cookie batter onto the cookie sheets in little mounds. These cookies won't rise or spread.

8. Bake in the preheated oven for approx. 20–25 mins or until the cookies are cooked through and the bottoms are lightly golden brown.

9. Enjoy warm or at room temperature.

The Solar Plexus Chakra

Yellow foods are vibrant in color and perfect for supporting solar plexus chakra balance. Yellow is also great for naturally improving your mood. Think of yellow fruits and vegetables, such as bananas, pineapple, lemons, and corn (non-GMO), that can be put into recipes or eaten on their own.

Complex carbohydrates and whole grains are fantastic for a slow release of energy and fiber, so include ingredients like brown rice, farro, beans, sprouted grains, and oats for easy meal prep items that can be combined with lots of different ingredients for healthy meal ideas.

Overnight Oats with Banana, Nut Butter, and Cinnamon

Servings: 2 people

Ingredients

½ cup gluten free oats or old-fashioned oats

1 serving vanilla protein powder

1 ripe banana

1 tsp ground cinnamon

1 Tbsp stevia or monk fruit sweetener, optional

1 ½–2 cups of water or milk of your choice

Toppings

1 Tbsp of nut butter of your choice, dash of cinnamon, berries of your choice

Instructions

1. In a medium-sized bowl, mash the banana until smooth.

2. Add the oats, vanilla protein powder, and ground cinnamon. Mix thoroughly. If your protein powder is not very sweet, you may also want to add the stevia or monk fruit sweetener.

3. Gradually pour in the water or milk of your choice and slowly stir to incorporate into the oat mixture.

4. Transfer the mixture into two resealable containers.

5. Cover the containers—or if they have lids, place the lids on the containers—and place in the fridge overnight. This will allow the oats to soak up the water or the milk of your choice and become tender.

6. Before serving the next day, drizzle over about 1 Tbsp of nut butter per serving, an extra dash of cinnamon, and some fresh berries too.

Grilled Hawaiian Chicken Skewers with Pineapple and Bell Peppers

Servings: 4 people

Ingredients

1 cup sugar-free BBQ sauce
¼ cup pineapple juice
1 Tbsp organic non-GMO soy sauce or coconut aminos
2 cloves garlic, minced
¼ cup cilantro, roughly chopped
1" piece of fresh ginger, grated
¼ tsp black pepper
2 lbs chicken breast, cut into 1" cubes
2 orange bell peppers, cut into 1" pieces
1 pineapple, cut into 1" pieces

Instructions

1. In a small bowl, mix together the BBQ sauce, pineapple juice, soy sauce/coconut aminos, cilantro, ginger, garlic, and black pepper.

2. Transfer half of the marinade into a large resealable bag and add the chicken pieces. Seal the bag and place in the fridge to marinate for at least 1 hour or overnight. Reserve the remaining marinade and place in the fridge.

3. While the chicken is marinating, soak your bamboo skewers in water for approximately 30 minutes.

4. When the chicken is done marinating, skewer alternating pieces of chicken, bell peppers, and pineapple until your skewers are about ¾ full. Repeat with remaining skewers. Discard the marinade that the chicken was in.

5. Grill the chicken skewers about 5 minutes per side, basting a couple of times with the reserved marinade. Once fully cooked, serve warm with your favorite sides!

Stir-fried Green Beans and Tofu with Yellow Coconut Rice

Servings: 4 people

Ingredients

For the Yellow Coconut Rice

2 cups basmati rice

2 cups water

2 cups coconut milk

2 tsp ground turmeric

1 tsp ginger

1 stalk of lemongrass, approx 4" in length

1 tsp black pepper

For the Stir-fried Green Beans and Tofu

1 Tbsp avocado oil

1 onion, diced

1 lb green beans, stem ends trimmed

1 lb hard tofu, drained and cut into bite sized pieces

2 cloves of garlic, minced

1 Tbsp toasted sesame oil

1 tsp salt

½ tsp black pepper

Ingredients

1. For the rice, place the rice in a fine mesh sieve and rinse under running water to help to remove some of the starches. Stop rinsing when the water coming out of the bottom of the sieve is almost clear.

2. Transfer the rice to a large pot that has a lid. Add the water, coconut milk, turmeric, ginger and black pepper. Stir well.

3. Take the lemongrass stalk, place it on a cutting board, then using the back of a chef's knife, hit the lemongrass stalk to start to break it open, but don't break or cut it open. Place the lemongrass into the pot with the rice. Stir once more.

4. Cover the pot and place it on the stovetop on high heat. Bring the rice to a boil, then reduce the heat to low and simmer until all the liquid has been absorbed.

5. Allow the rice to sit and stay warm while you make the Stir Fried Green Beans and Tofu.

6. For the Stir-fried Green Beans and Tofu, take a large sauté pan or wok and heat over high heat. Add the avocado oil.

7. Once the oil is hot, add the onion and stir-fry for about 1-2 minutes or until the onion is slightly translucent and the edges are starting to brown.

8. Add the green beans and stir-fry with the onions, stirring frequently for about 5 minutes, until the green beans are starting to become tender.

9. Add the garlic cloves and stir continuously as it becomes fragrant.

10. Add the tofu pieces and stir quickly into the vegetable mixture.

11. Turn the heat off and add the sesame oil, salt, and pepper. Stir quickly to incorporate into the mixture and coat all the veggies and tofu.

12. To serve, add about a ½ cup portion of rice to a plate and add the Stir Fried Green Beans and Tofu to the side. Enjoy immediately!

Air-fried Chickpeas with Turmeric and Paprika

Servings: 4 people

Ingredients

1 can chickpeas, rinsed and drained
1 tsp avocado oil
½ tsp ground turmeric
½ tsp ground paprika
½ tsp salt
¼ tsp finely ground black pepper

Instructions

1. Take the rinsed and drained chickpeas and place them on a kitchen towel or some paper towels. Thoroughly dry the chickpeas. This may take off the top layer of the skin of the chickpeas and that is totally ok!

2. Transfer the chickpeas to a medium-sized bowl, then add the oil, turmeric, paprika, salt, and pepper. Stir well to coat the chickpeas evenly with the seasonings and oil.

3. Pour the seasoned chickpeas into the basket of your air fryer.

4. Roast the chickpeas in the air fryer at 380°F for 12-15 minutes, shaking the basket every 5 minutes or so to prevent any burning or uneven cooking. Cook until the chickpeas are golden brown and crispy.

5. Serve the chickpeas as a snack or a great topping for a salad too.

Easy Mango, Peppers, and Black Bean Salsa

Servings: 4 people

Ingredients

1 large mango, peeled and diced into small pieces

1 yellow banana pepper, halved lengthwise and cut into small pieces

1 jalapeno, stems and seeds removed to reduce the heat if desired and cut into small pieces

¼ cup yellow bell pepper, diced into small pieces

¼ cup orange bell pepper, diced into small pieces

1 large lime

½ cup fresh cilantro, roughly chopped

¼ cup red onion, finely diced

½ cup black beans, washed, rinsed, and dried

1 tsp salt

½ tsp black pepper

Instructions

1. In a medium-sized bowl, add the mango pieces, banana pepper, jalapeno, yellow and orange bell peppers, zest and juice of the lime, cilantro, red onion, black beans, salt, and pepper.

2. Stir well to fully incorporate.

3. Taste and see if additional salt and pepper is needed.

4. Serve with your favorite chips or crackers or use this salsa to top tacos or salads.

"Don't overlook your greatest healing tool... Your Intuition."

– CAROLYN HARRINGTON

The Heart Chakra

Green foods are fantastic for supporting the heart center. I love to incorporate kale, spinach, broccoli, cucumber, zucchini, and all kinds of peas in my weekly meals. Other ingredients you can try are green apples, kiwi fruit, avocado, parsley, celery, cilantro, and even spirulina, which is a powerful superfood packed with nutrients including protein, iron, vitamins B1, B2, and B3.

Typically, raw green foods are recommended for this chakra. However, some people may find it challenging at first to digest so many additional green vegetables and fruits. This is usually because raw foods require the body to work a little harder to digest or break down the fruits and vegetables. Some ways to mitigate this include a gradual increase over time in the amount of raw foods you consume or having mostly cooked greens and then slowly transition to more raw greens. Both of these methods allow the body to slowly be able to consume more raw greens, lessening the discomfort that may accompany a big shift in diet.

Green tea and matcha are two drinks that are powerful for supporting the heart space and also have scientifically proven benefits such as reducing inflammation, improved brain function, and protecting against the risk of heart disease. You can also get a boost of greens from green juices or smoothies. I prefer smoothies because of the increased fiber content vs most green juices. There is a recipe below for an easy, fiber-packed green smoothie you can add green herbs and spirulina to for the ultimate heart chakra smoothie.

HEART CHAKRA RECIPES

The Ultimate Heart Chakra Smoothie

Servings: 1 person

Ingredients

1 Tbsp chia seeds

1 Tbsp flax seeds

1 tsp green spirulina

1 small green apple, chopped

2 cups kale or spinach leaves

1 cup cucumber

2 stalks celery, chopped

¼ fresh or frozen avocado

1 serving of collagen powder of your choice

½ lemon, juiced

1 cup ice

1–2 cups water, depending on desired consistency

Instructions

1. To a high-speed blender, add all the ingredients. Add more water if you prefer a thinner consistency to your smoothie.

2. Place the lid on the blender and blend until the smoothie is nice and creamy.

3. Serve immediately!

Kale Taco Salad

Servings: 4 people

Ingredients

1 tsp avocado oil
1 onion, diced
2 lb ground turkey
1 Tbsp chili powder
1 ½ tsp cumin
1 tsp dried oregano
½ tsp black pepper
1 tsp garlic powder

For the Salad

8 cups of baby kale
1 cup black beans, rinsed and drained
½ cup cherry tomatoes, halved
½ cup queso fresco, crumbled
1 avocado, diced
1 large lime, quartered
4 tsp roasted pepitas or pumpkin seeds
1 ½ cups of your favorite salsa

Instructions

1. Heat a large sauté pan over medium heat. Add the oil.

2. Once the oil is hot, add the ground turkey and cook over medium heat, breaking up the meat occasionally with a wooden spoon until the turkey is completely cooked through.

3. Add the onion, and continue to sauté until the onion is softened, about another 5 minutes.

4. Add the remaining seasonings to the pan and stir thoroughly to incorporate it into the ground turkey and onion mixture.

5. On each plate, add 2 cups of baby kale in a single layer.

6. Top with the cooked turkey taco meat, then scatter the black beans, cherry tomatoes, queso fresco, avocado, and pumpkin seeds over the kale as well.

7. Take one quarter of the lime and squeeze over the salad. Add your favorite salsa as a final topping before enjoying!

Cucumber-Mint Infused Coconut Water

Servings: 4 people

Ingredients

4 cups coconut water
4 cups water
1 cucumber, sliced into thin rounds
1 cup fresh mint, leaves picked off the stem
Ice

Instructions

1. To a large 10–12-cup pitcher, add the coconut water and water. Stir to combine.

2. Add cucumber slices and fresh mint leaves, as much as the pitcher will hold, and stir once more to submerge the cucumber slices. Allow the mint leaves to start to bruise a little so that the essential oils are released.

3. Top with ice or place the pitcher in the fridge to chill.

4. Serve in tall glasses with more ice if desired.

Roasted Broccoli Salad
with a Green Goddess Dressing

Servings: 4 people

Ingredients

2 large heads of broccoli
1 large sweet onion
1 Tbsp avocado oil
1 tsp salt
1 tsp black pepper

For the Green Goddess Dressing

1 cup low-fat Greek yogurt or an unflavored yogurt of your
   choice
1 cup fresh parsley
½ cup fresh cilantro
¼ cup fresh dill leaves
¼ cup fresh mint leaves
2 Tbsp green onions or chives, chopped
1 large lemon, zested and juiced
1 Tbsp extra virgin olive oil
2 tsp capers
1 garlic clove
¼ tsp sea salt
⅛ tsp black pepper

Instructions

1. Preheat the oven to 420°F.

2. Cut large florets off of the broccoli heads.

3. Chop the stems into bite-sized pieces.

4. Transfer the broccoli to a large rimmed baking sheet.

5. Drizzle over the olive oil, salt, and pepper, then toss together to fully incorporate.

6. Ensure the broccoli is in an even layer on the baking sheet, then place in the preheated oven.

7. Roast for about 20 mins or until the broccoli is crisp on the edges and the stalk is tender.

8. Meanwhile, for the Green Goddess dressing, add all ingredients into a blender or food processor. Blend until smooth.

9. Taste and see if any additional seasonings are needed.

10. To serve, transfer the broccoli to a plate and pour over the Green Goddess dressing.

Continue connecting
with your chakras
by downloading
the meditations at
http://www.
nourishwithrenata.com/
healyourbodymind
andspirit

Air Fryer Broccolini with Creamy Scrambled Eggs

Servings: 2 people

Ingredients

1 Tbsp grass-fed butter
4 eggs
2 Tbsp water or milk of your choice
1 tsp salt
½ tsp black pepper
1 large bunch of broccolini, washed and dried well
1 tsp avocado oil
½ tsp salt
¼ tsp black pepper

Instructions

1. To a medium-sized bowl, add the eggs, water (or milk) salt, and pepper. Whisk together very well to fully blend the eggs together.

2. Heat a large nonstick pan over medium low heat. Add the butter.

3. Once the butter has melted, pour the egg mixture into the pan.

4. Cook the eggs over medium low heat, stirring occasionally with a spatula or wooden spoon to carefully move around and break up the eggs. Cooking the eggs at a low temperature for a longer amount of time results in creamy scrambled eggs. Continue doing this until the eggs are fully cooked and still soft and creamy.

5. Meanwhile, trim the very ends of the broccolini stalks to remove any particular dry or hard areas. Make sure the length of the broccolini will fit into your air fryer and if not, trim more of the ends or cut the broccolini into appropriately sized pieces.

6. Add the broccolini to a medium-sized bowl and add the oil, salt, and pepper. Toss well to evenly coat the broccolini with the oil and seasonings.

7. Transfer the broccolini to the basket of your air fryer. Cook the broccolini in the air fryer at 375°F for about 7-9 minutes, or until the broccolini is bright green and tender crisp.

8. To serve, add half of the air fryer broccolini to a plate, then pair with the creamy scrambled eggs alongside. Enjoy immediately!

The Throat Chakra

This chakra can be supported with blue foods such as blueberries and blackberries. These berries are low in natural sugars while also being high in antioxidants, vitamins, and fiber. In addition, the throat chakra, being related to the voice box and physiological throat, benefits from hydration and soothing drinks like water, coconut water, and decaffeinated herbal teas with raw honey and lemon.

THROAT CHAKRA RECIPES

Blueberry Nice Cream with Honey and Mint

Servings: 2 people

Ingredients

1 banana, sliced into pieces and frozen
1 cup frozen blueberries
1–2 Tbsp of milk of choice, optional
1 Tbsp local honey + extra for garnish
1 Tbsp fresh mint leaves

Instructions

1. In a blender, add the banana, blueberries, and honey.

2. Place the lid on the blender. If you have a tamper device, you will want to insert this into the lid of the blender or be ready to scrape the inside of the blender several times during the next phase.

3. Carefully blend the banana, blueberries, and honey, using the tamper to push the frozen ingredients towards the blade or stop the blender and use a spatula to scrape the insides of the blender to reincorporate the ingredients. Continue doing so until a creamy ice cream texture is achieved. You may also want to add a little milk to the blender in case the mixture is too thick and you desire a creamier consistency.

4. Transfer the Blueberry Nice Cream to two bowls, top with an extra drizzle of honey and some fresh torn mint leaves.

5. Serve immediately!

Frozen Yogurt Blueberry and Orange Bites

Servings: 4 people

Ingredients

1 pint fresh blueberries, washed and dried
1 Tbsp fresh orange zest
2 cups low-fat Greek yogurt, vanilla or unflavored

Instructions

1. To a medium-sized bowl, add the blueberries, orange zest, and the yogurt. Mix well to fully coat the blueberries with the yogurt and evenly distribute the orange zest.

2. Take an oven tray and line with a nonstick mat or parchment paper.

3. Scoop tablespoons of the yogurt-blueberry mixture onto the tray. You can place each tablespoon of the mixture about ½ inch apart.

4. Transfer the tray to the freezer and freeze until completely set and hardened.

5. Enjoy these Frozen Yogurt Blueberry and Orange Bites as a refreshing snack straight from the freezer or wait a couple minutes to allow them to soften slightly before eating.

Blackberry and Peach Crumble

Servings: 4 people

Ingredients

2 pints of blackberries, washed

2 large peaches, washed & chopped into bite-sized pieces

1–2 Tbsp of stevia or monk fruit sweetener, depending on
the sweetness of your berries and peaches

1 tsp vanilla extract

1 tsp ground cinnamon

For the Crumble Topping

2 Tbsp coconut oil, melted

2 Tbsp sweetener of your choice, like stevia

½ cup gluten-free oats

½ cup pecan pieces

Instructions

1. Preheat the oven to 350°F.

2. To a large bowl, add the blackberries, chopped peaches, stevia or monk fruit sweetener, vanilla extract, and cinnamon. Toss together to combine evenly, then transfer the fruit mixture to an oven-safe pie dish.

3. In a medium-sized bowl, add the oats, pecans, sweetener, and coconut oil. Stir together until the mixture creates a crumbly texture.

4. Sprinkle this crumble evenly over the blackberries and peaches.

5. Bake in a preheated oven for about 30 minutes or until the peaches are softened, the blackberries are releasing their beautiful ruby juices, and the crumble is golden brown.

6. Serve with your favorite vanilla ice cream or frozen yogurt.

Blueberry, Blackberry, and Lime Chia Seed Jam

Servings: 8 people

Ingredients

1 pint of blueberries, washed
1 pint of blackberries, washed
1 large lime, zested and juiced
2 Tbsp chia seeds
2 Tbsp stevia or monk fruit sweetener

Instructions

1. Place the berries in a small pot and add the lime juice and sweetener.

2. Heat the pot over medium heat, stirring occasionally as the heat allows the berries to burst and their juices to be released.

3. Once the berries are fully softened and there is a lot of moisture in the pot, turn off the heat and add the chia seeds. Stir well to fully combine.

4. Remove the pot from the heat and add the lime zest. Stir once more.

5. Allow the mixture to cool, then taste and see if additional sweetener is required.

6. Transfer the jam to jars with a tight-fitting lid. Keep in the fridge for up 2–3 weeks. Serve with biscuits, toast, or on protein oatmeal.

Blackberry Quinoa Salad with a Citrus Olive Oil Dressing

Servings: 4 people

Ingredients

1 cup quinoa

2 cups water

1 pint blackberries, washed

1 nectarine, cut into thin wedges

½ red onion, finely sliced

2 cups of arugula or other greens of your choice

For the Citrus Olive Oil Dressing

1 mandarin orange, zested and juiced

1 lemon, zested and juiced

1 lime, zested and juiced

1 Tbsp stevia or monk fruit sweetener

1 garlic clove, minced

½ cup extra virgin olive oil

1 tsp salt

½ tsp black pepper

Instructions

1. To cook the quinoa, add the quinoa and water to a medium-sized pot. Place a lid on the pot and cook over medium heat.

2. Bring the mixture to a boil, then reduce to a simmer, keeping the lid on. Continue to cook the quinoa until all the liquid is absorbed, about 10 minutes.

3. Cool the quinoa.

4. Meanwhile, add all the ingredients for the Citrus Olive Oil Dressing into a jar with a tight-fitting lid. Screw the lid on the jar and shake the jar vigorously to fully incorporate the dressing ingredients. Set aside until ready to use.

5. Once the quinoa is cooled, add the quinoa to a large bowl. Top with the arugula or other greens, red onion slices, wedges of nectarine, and the blackberries.

6. Shake the dressing jar once again to mix up the ingredients, and pour about ½ a cup of the dressing over the salad.

7. Toss the quinoa salad to combine all the ingredients with the dressing and evenly distribute the blackberries, nectarines, greens, and red onion.

8. Serve the salad alongside your favorite protein of choice.

Ask yourself:
"What is one thing
I can do right now
to connect more deeply
with my body, mind,
and spirit?"

The Third Eye Chakra

Purple foods are fantastic for supporting this chakra. Consider incorporating foods like eggplant, purple cabbage, grapes, and purple carrots. Not only are they a great source of vitamins and minerals, these fruits and vegetables are a great source of fiber, which is so important for overall gut health. Since there is a link between the gut and the brain, having a healthy gut is really important to help support brain health as well as third eye chakra health.

Once again, a good quality dark chocolate, or more specifically cacao, is wonderful for this chakra, as well as the sacral chakra. Dark chocolate, or cacao, helps reduce inflammation due to the antioxidants, and can increase your mood regulating neurotransmitter, serotonin. In fact, about 80–90% of serotonin is created in the gut which then has a direct impact on the brain and also the third eye chakra.

Chocolate Superfood Protein Balls

Servings: 10 protein balls

Ingredients

⅔ cup gluten free oats

¾ cup sugar free almond butter

1 serving of vanilla protein powder + extra if your mixture is
  too soft

1 tsp vanilla extract

1 Tbsp chia seeds

1 Tbsp flax seeds

¼ cup pumpkin seeds

¼ cup sesame seeds

¼ cup sunflower seeds

2 Tbsp cocoa powder

Instructions

1. To a medium-sized bowl, add all the ingredients. Mix
   thoroughly to fully incorporate.

2. If your mixture is too soft, add a little more protein
   powder, one tablespoon at a time until the mixture holds
   together when pressed into a ball.

3. Take tablespoons of the mixture and create protein
   balls, rolling them in between the palms of your hands.
   Continue doing so until all of the protein mixture has
   been used up.

4. Place the protein balls in an airtight container and keep
   in the fridge for up to one week.

Rainbow Salad with Purple Kale

Servings: 4 people

Ingredients

4 cups purple kale, finely sliced

2 cups grated carrots

1 yellow bell peppers, chopped into small pieces

1 cup cherry tomatoes, halved

1 avocado, sliced

1 cup cucumber, diced

1 cup blueberries, washed and dried

For the easy Creamy Lemon Dressing

1 Tbsp mayonnaise of your choice

1 lemon, zested and juiced

¼ cup extra virgin olive oil

1 tbsp stevia, monk fruit sweetener, or honey

1 tsp salt

½ tsp black pepper

Instructions

1. For the Creamy Lemon Dressing, add all the ingredients into a jar with a tight-fitting lid.

2. Screw the lid on the jar and shake vigorously to fully incorporate and emulsify the ingredients. Set aside while you assemble the Rainbow Salad.

3. For the salad, take a large serving bowl and add a bed of the purple kale.

4. Top the purple kale with each of the remaining ingredients in colorful mounds.

5. Drizzle over some of the Creamy Lemon Dressing.

6. Serve immediately!

Purple Carrot Carpaccio

Servings: 2 people

Ingredients

1 large orange carrot
1 large yellow carrot
2 large purple carrots
¼ cup extra virgin olive oil
4 Tbsp white wine vinegar
½ cup cherry tomatoes, any color, halved
1 Tbsp fresh basil leaves
1 Tbsp fresh oregano leaves
1 Tbsp toasted pine nuts
Sprinkle of sea salt
Finely ground black pepper

Instructions

1. Carefully using a mandolin, finely slice the carrots into super thin rounds.

2. Place these rounds into a large bowl.

3. Add the extra virgin olive oil and white wine vinegar. Stir well then allow to sit for about 1 hour to soften the carrots.

4. After an hour, take the carrot slices and place on a serving plate.

5. Scatter over the cherry tomatoes then tear over the basil and oregano leaves.

6. Finally, top with the pine nuts and a pinch of sea salt and finely ground black pepper.

7. Enjoy immediately!

Roasted Purple Cabbage with Creamy Cilantro Lime Dressing

Servings: 4 people

Ingredients

1 head of purple cabbage
1 Tbsp avocado oil
1 tsp ground cumin
1 tsp salt
1 tsp black pepper

For the Creamy Cilantro Lime Dressing

¼ cup olive oil
¼ cup mayonnaise of your choice
1 large bunch of fresh cilantro
2 large limes, zested and juiced
1 tsp salt
½ tsp black pepper

Instructions

1. Preheat the oven to 425°F.

2. Quarter the purple cabbage, then cut the core out of each wedge.

3. Slice the cabbage into slices about ½ inch thick.

4. Transfer the cabbage to 1 or 2 large rimmed baking sheets.

5. Drizzle with avocado oil, then season with cumin, salt, and pepper.

6. Roast in a preheated oven for about 15–20 minutes or until the cabbage is slightly tender and the edges are crisp and golden.

7. Meanwhile for the Creamy Cilantro Lime Dressing, add all the ingredients to a blender and blend until smooth. Taste and adjust seasonings as desired.

8. To serve, place some of the roasted purple cabbage on a plate, and drizzle over about 1 Tbsp of the Creamy Cilantro Lime Dressing. Enjoy immediately!

Roasted Eggplant with Spicy Chili Sauce

Servings: 4 people

Ingredients

2 large eggplants, washed and sliced into 1" thick rounds
1 Tbsp avocado oil
1 tsp salt
½ tsp black pepper

For the Spicy Chili Sauce

2 Tbsp avocado oil
1 large onion, finely chopped
1 large tomato, finely chopped
2 cloves of garlic, minced
1 Tbsp lemon juice
1 Tbsp stevia or monk fruit sweetener
1 Tbsp red pepper flakes
1 Tbsp chipotle powder
1 Tbsp ground spicy chilies such as Thai red chili powder
1 tsp salt

Instructions

1. Preheat the oven to 425°F.

2. Take 2 large rimmed baking trays and place the eggplant rounds on the trays in a single layer.

3. Drizzle over the avocado oil, salt, and pepper and rub into each of the eggplant slices.

4. Roast the eggplant in a preheated oven for about 15 minutes. Carefully turn over each eggplant slice and roast for another 15 minutes or until the eggplant is tender and golden.

5. Meanwhile, heat a large sauté pan over medium heat.

6. Add the avocado oil to the pan and when warm, add the onion.

7. Sauté the onion until softened, about 5 minutes.

8. Add the tomato and continue to cook for another 5 minutes to break down the tomatoes.

9. Add the garlic, and stir until fragrant, about 1 minute.

10. Add the lemon juice, stevia, or monk fruit sweetener, red pepper flakes, chipotle powder, ground chilies, and salt. Stir very well to fully combine the ingredients.

11. Continue to sauté the tomato, onion, and chili mixture for another 5-10 minutes until it is a deep, rich, red color and the onions and tomatoes have almost fully broken down.

12. To serve, add a few eggplant slices to a plate and top with 1-2 Tbsp of the chili sauce. Enjoy immediately!

Note: Store any remaining Spicy Chili Sauce in an airtight container in the fridge for up to 2 weeks.

The Crown Chakra

The crown chakra is supported by detoxification of the body as well as the alignment and balance of the rest of the chakras. This helps to open up the crown chakra and allow for the spiritual connection to our bodies and minds. Detoxification can happen in many ways, such as by increasing water intake, reducing toxins from the environment, and foods and eating fiber-rich foods to aid the natural detoxification process. In particular, cruciferous vegetables, such as cabbage, kale, broccoli and cauliflower, contain a compound called IC3 that breaks down toxins in the body so that they can be eliminated through bowel movements. You can also eliminate or at least reduce alcohol, excessively caffeinated beverages, refined sugar, and processed foods during the detox period you choose or start instilling this in your daily routine to create a sustainable, healthier lifestyle.

There are some great herbs or essential oils that can help support the crown chakra such as lavender, sage, frankincense and juniper. These herbs can be added to meals or you can diffuse these essential oils in your house.

In addition to food, experimenting or embracing some spiritual techniques described in this section (such as meditation and breathwork) can be very helpful for continuing to strengthen your crown chakra. Taking time to be mindful each and every day is a powerful practice energetically as well as having a positive impact on your physical wellbeing too.

CROWN CHAKRA RECIPES

Easy Crockpot Bone Broth

Ingredients

Bones from 2 roasted chickens or 1 turkey

2 stalks celery, cut into thirds

1 yellow onion, cut in quarters

2 medium carrots, cut in half

4 cloves garlic

2 tsp ground turmeric

1 3-inch piece ginger, sliced

1 Tbsp apple cider vinegar

10 cups water (or enough to cover all the ingredients)

2 tsp kosher salt

10 black peppercorns

2 bay leaves

Instructions

1. Add all the ingredients into your crockpot insert, making sure you add enough water to cover all the ingredients.

2. Place the lid on the crockpot and cook over medium heat for about 12 hours or low heat for about 18 hours. You can even cook for as long as 24 hours. You want the broth to look rich in color and for the vegetables to have broken down in the broth. You can also skim the top of the broth occasionally to remove any impurities or fats that are collecting on the surface of the bone broth.

3. Carefully strain the broth through a fine mesh strainer to ensure that any little bits from the vegetables and bones do not end up in the final bone broth.

4. Taste to see if the broth needs more salt and add as desired.

5. Allow the broth to cool and transfer it to jars or resealable containers.

6. Keep in the fridge if using in soups, stews or planning to sip on the broth during the day. Alternatively, freeze the bone broth to be used later. Make sure to leave enough room in the glass jar or container so that there is space for the liquid to expand as it freezes.

Simple Crunchy Cabbage Salad

Servings: 4 people

Ingredients

½ head of green cabbage, finely sliced
½ head of purple cabbage, finely sliced
1 large bunch of cilantro, roughly chopped
½ red onion, finely sliced
¼ cup toasted almond slivers
¼ cup toasted pepitas or pumpkin seeds

For the Dressing

¼ cup olive oil
2 large lemons, juiced
2 tsp salt
1 tsp black pepper

Instructions

1. To a very large bowl, add the green and purple cabbage slices.

2. Add the cilantro and red onion, then toss all the vegetables together to evenly distribute.

3. For the dressing, add all the ingredients into a jar with a tight-fitting lid.

4. Screw the lid on the jar and shake vigorously to combine.

5. Pour half of the dressing over the cabbage mixture and toss well. If needed, add more of the dressing and toss again.

6. Before serving, scatter the toasted almonds and pumpkin seeds over the cabbage salad.

7. Enjoy immediately!

Kale and Lemon Detox Smoothie

Servings: 1 person

Ingredients

1 Tbsp chia seeds

2 cups kale

1 x 1-inch piece of fresh ginger, skin removed and chopped into smaller pieces

1 lemon, juiced

1 serving collagen powder

1 tsp spirulina

1–2 cups water

1 cup ice

Instructions

1. Add all ingredients into a blender and blend until super smooth. Add more water if you desire a thinner consistency or add more ice if you like it to be colder and thicker.

2. Enjoy immediately!

Chlorella Water

Servings: 1 person

Ingredients

1 tsp chlorella powder
16 oz water or coconut water
Optional: ice, lemon slices

Instructions

1. Add chlorella powder to a glass.

2. Add about 2 oz of water and mix well with the chlorella to fully dissolve.

3. Top with the remaining water and some ice or lemon slices if desired.

Turmeric, Ginger and Lemon Wellness Shots

Servings: 2 people

Ingredients

1 small orange, juiced
1 lemon, juiced
¼ inch piece of turmeric root
¼ inch piece of ginger
Pinch of black pepper
½ tsp coconut oil
¼ cup of water, if needed

Instructions

1. In a blender, add the orange juice, lemon juice, turmeric, and ginger roots, pinch of black pepper, and oil.

2. Blend to create a super smooth mixture, adding some water if needed to fully incorporate all the ingredients if they are stuck to the insides of the blender.

3. You can choose if you'd like to strain the wellness shots through a cheesecloth or very fine mesh sieve, or enjoy the pulp in the wellness shot.

4. Divide the wellness shots between two glasses and enjoy immediately.

"We are not our thoughts.
We are the observer
of the thoughts.
We are not our beliefs.
We are the consciousness
that observes those
beliefs."

– RENATA TREBING

RECIPES FOR ALL THE CHAKRAS

One of my favorite things to do is incorporate lots of color into my recipes. Not only is this visually appealing, but it also helps to support all the chakras in one meal. Here are some of my favorite recipes that use food to support all of the seven main chakras.

Shrimp Nourish Bowls with Roasted Vegetables, Black Beans, and Mango Salsa

Servings: 4 people

Ingredients

For the Cilantro Lime Rice

2 cups rice of your choice e.g. white rice, brown rice.
4 cups water
1 cup cilantro, chopped
2 large limes, juiced and zested

For the Roasted Vegetables

1 large onion, chopped into large chunks
2 bell peppers, sliced into 1/2-inch-thick strips
2 zucchinis, chopped into large chunks
1 Tbsp olive oil
1 tsp salt
½ tsp black pepper

For the Mango Salsa

1 large mango, diced
1 lime, halved
¼ cup fresh cilantro, chopped
½ tsp salt

For the Black Beans

1 can of black beans, drained, rinsed, and dried
1/3 cup fresh cilantro, chopped
¼ cup white onion, finely chopped
1 tsp salt
½ tsp black pepper

For the Chipotle Shrimp

2 lbs shrimp, peeled and deveined
2 tsp avocado oil
2 tsp chipotle powder

Instructions

For the Cilantro Lime Rice

1. Rinse the rice in running water to help remove some of the sticky starches.

2. In a large pot with a tight-fitting lid, add the rice and the water.

3. Place the pot over high heat to bring to the boil with the lid on. Once boiling, reduce the heat to low and allow to simmer until the rice is completely cooked through, about 20 minutes for white rice or 45 minutes for brown rice.

4. Stir the rice to fluff it up.

5. Add the lime juice, zest, and cilantro.

6. Toss together to combine well.

7. Set aside until ready to serve.

For the Roasted Vegetables

1. Preheat the oven to 400°F.

2. On a large rimmed baking sheet, add the onion, bell peppers, and zucchini.

3. Drizzle over the olive oil, salt, and pepper and toss to combine.

4. Roast in the preheated oven for about 30 minutes, tossing them halfway through the cooking time. Aim for the vegetables to be tender and caramelized at the edges.

5. Keep warm until ready to serve.

For the Mango Salsa

1. In a medium-sized bowl, add the mango, fresh cilantro, and salt. Squeeze in the lime juice.

2. Toss together to combine.

3. Set aside until ready to serve.

For the Black Beans

1. In a medium-sized bowl, add the black beans, onions, fresh cilantro, salt, and pepper.

2. Toss together to combine.

3. Set aside until ready to serve.

For the Chipotle Shrimp

1. Preheat a large sauté pan over medium high heat.

2. Add the oil.

3. Once the oil is hot, add the shrimp in a single layer (you may need to do this in multiple batches).

4. Cook the shrimp for about 2-3 minutes, or until the underside is golden brown.

5. Turn the shrimp carefully to cook on the second side for approximately 2-3 minutes again.

6. Sprinkle on the chipotle powder to season the shrimp. **Note:** This could create a strong chili scent in the air, which will be great for opening the throat chakra!

7. Remove the cooked shrimp from the pan and place on a plate to keep warm.

8. Repeat the last four steps with any remaining shrimp.

9. To serve, add a bed of cilantro lime rice. Top with the roasted veggies, black beans, mango salsa, and the chipotle shrimp. Enjoy!

Moroccan Roasted Vegetable Salad with a Citrus Tahini Dressing

Servings: 4 people

Ingredients

For the Citrus Tahini Dressing

¼ cup tahini
¼ cup fresh orange juice + ½ tsp orange zest
2 Tablespoons apple cider vinegar
1-2 tsp stevia or monk fruit sweetener
2 tsp minced garlic
2 tsp Dijon mustard
¼ tsp salt
1–2 Tbsps water, if necessary

For the Moroccan Roasted Vegetable Salad

2 large onions, roughly chopped
2 large sweet potatoes, chopped into bite-sized pieces
2 large red or yellow bell peppers, cut into ½-inch-thick strips
2 large zucchinis, chopped into large chunks
2 Tbsps olive oil + 1 tsp olive oil
2 tsp ground cumin
1 tsp ground coriander
½ tsp ground cinnamon
2 tsp salt
1 tsp black pepper
8 cups of kale
1 can chickpeas, drained and rinsed

Instructions

For the Citrus Tahini Dressing

1. Add all ingredients, except the water, into a large jar that has a tight-fitting lid.

2. Tighten the lid on the jar and shake the jar vigorously to combine all of the ingredients.

3. If the dressing is too thick for your liking, add the water and shake the dressing again to combine.

4. Store the dressing in the fridge for up to one week. You can also make this dressing ahead of time prior to serving the salad.

For the Moroccan Roasted Vegetable Salad

1. Preheat the oven to 400°F.

2. Take 2 large rimmed baking trays and evenly distribute the onions, sweet potatoes, bell peppers, and zucchini.

3. Drizzle 1 Tbsp of olive oil over the veggies in each pan.

4. Season the vegetables with the cumin, coriander, cinnamon, salt, and pepper. Toss together to evenly coat the veggies.

5. Roast the vegetables in the preheated oven for approximately 40 minutes, stirring halfway through the cooking time. Aim to have the vegetables caramelized on the edges and tender.

6. Meanwhile, heat a large sauté pan over medium heat.

7. Add 1 tsp olive oil then add the kale.

8. Sauté the kale until softened, about 8-10 minutes, stirring frequently.

9. Add the chickpeas. Toss together to combine.

10. Season with salt and pepper as desired.

11. To serve, add some of the kale and chickpea mixture to a plate, top with the roasted vegetables, then drizzle over the Citrus Tahini dressing.

Rainbow Stir-fry for the Chakras

Servings: 4 people

Ingredients

1 lb chicken breast, sliced thinly

1 onion, cut into eighths

1 head broccoli, cut into florets

2 cups sliced carrots

2 cups purple cabbage, finely sliced

1 red bell pepper, finely sliced

1 yellow bell pepper, finely sliced

1 cup snow peas

2 cloves garlic, finely sliced

For the Sauce

$1/3$ cup light soy sauce or coconut aminos

$1/3$ cup water

3 Tbsp stevia or monk fruit sweetener

1 tsp ground ginger

1 tsp garlic powder or 1 fresh garlic clove, minced

Instructions

1. In a large saucepan or wok on medium high heat, cook the sliced chicken until cooked through.

2. In a small bowl, mix together all the sauce ingredients.

3. Increase the heat for the pan/wok to high, then add in all the vegetables and sauce.

4. Stir-fry all the ingredients, stirring frequently, so that the sauce has coated all of the ingredients and the veggies are crisp tender.

Energetic Transfer and Leaks

Our body's energy can influence the people around us, and the opposite is true too. Other people's energy can influence our energy.

This is great when the people we are surrounded by are positive and uplifting people. However, if you are around negative influences, it can be very easy for those qualities to start to affect you too, often without you even realizing it for some time.

Awareness is always the key before any change can be made. Periodically check in with your body and energy to see if you're feeling drained, reinvigorated, stressed, nervous, excited, joyful, etc. Make a mental note of how your energy feels without outside influence and how that energy changes as you are influenced by other people, places, and things. Understanding these energetic transfers is important because you will quickly become attuned to if your energy is being affected by others and if so, how to clear this energy from your electromagnetic field. I recommend going back to the Chakra Clearing Meditation on a regular basis to help keep you aligned and your energy free from outside influences as much as possible.

An energetic leak is when your energy is leaking from one particular or multiple chakras. This could feel like you are losing your self-confidence, your self-worth, or feeling completely doubtful about yourself and out of balance. An energetic leak is essentially giving your power away to someone or something else. Doing this for too long can cause habits that could potentially allow others to take advantage of you, or for emotional distress and physical disease to occur if the leak is not tended to and left to occur for a long duration of time.

Energetic leaks are another powerful realization because when you recognize that this is happening, you can tune into the chakras in question, and go through the Chakra Clearing meditation process above (see page 98) to clear and align your chakras so that you can get back into full alignment energetically.

You are a Powerful Being

Having shingles was a turning point in my deep understanding about healing the body. I truly believe that physical issues in the body occur after a long period of time where the emotional, mental, and energetic symptoms were not made aware of or healed. Instead, these negative thoughts and feelings cause negative actions to be made, such as not looking after yourself, which, when continued for a prolonged period, make it easier for physical disease to arise.

My healing from shingles then needed to occur on all levels of being.

Physically, I took the medicine from the doctor, ate healthfully, took supplements to improve my gut health and ensure I was having all the necessary vitamins and minerals. I rested and slept more than ever and removed as much stress as possible.

Energetically, I cleared my chakras, particularly my Root Chakra, the closest energy center to the shingles rash and pain. I also had to find ways to process challenging negative emotions, as well as coming back to breathwork and yoga.

Mentally, I had to recognize and release my negative thought patterns and limiting beliefs. Practicing mindfulness techniques like meditation and visualization helped immensely, especially with balancing my Root Chakra and visualizing the healing process occurring in my body.

Intuitively, I knew that I was not feeling grounded and stable (more root chakra work) and needed to have tough conversations to help the relationships that were causing me to feel off balance. I also used my intuitive senses to help me to figure out what my body needed at that moment.

Spiritually, I had to get back to my practices of mindfulness, honoring my connection to the Divine and using food to support my chakras and spiritual connection.

I'm happy to say that I have been completely shingles-free since this happened. I have not experienced the same level of stress, poor physical health, negativity or disconnectedness that I was feeling prior to being diagnosed, and I truly attribute this to understanding the powerful impact that healing on all levels can have on my wellness.

This all started with a choice.

A choice to confront the symptoms that I hadn't confronted before and be brutally honest with what was happening to me.

A choice to take the opportunity of having shingles and understanding healing on a deeper level.

A choice to heal my body, mind, and spirit no matter what.

You, too, have the power to heal your body, mind, and spirit. I hope that reading this book has shown you multiple different techniques, as well as the science and philosophy behind many of the holistic methodologies that I have seen has helped me in my own healing journey. I believe these methods will help you too.

Remember, you are a Powerful Being. You have the choice every single day to include one or more of these practices into your daily lifestyle.

Getting healthier and healing your body is not an overnight transformation. It is the culmination of daily practices, of daily habits, that allow you to slowly but surely shift from who you are now into who you ultimately want to be.

The choice is always yours.

Choose to be the most Powerful You there could be in this moment and every moment thereafter.

Choose to Heal.

Visit
http://www.
nourishwithrenata.com/
healyourbodymind
andspirit
for exclusive bonuses
and videos.

Acknowledgments

A huge thank you to my self-publishing mentor, Leesa Ellis of 3 ferns books. You are always so easy to work with, have such great ideas, and always go above and beyond. You make the book creation process so easy with your guidance and support. Thank you!

Thank you to my coach, Jacqueline Hopper, who kept telling me there was another book in me, that she knew what the topic was but she wouldn't tell me. She also said one day I would figure out the topic. I did it!

Thank you to my coach, Jessica Mclaren, for always listening deeply, asking profound questions and challenging me to BE all that I am. I am so inspired by you and the journey I have seen you live through. Thank you for being a stand for me and all the Next Level Life ladies. Huge shoutout to all the amazing women in the Next Level Life community too!

Thank you to all my incredible friends who are endless supporters, encouragers and advice-givers. Thank you Anne Laguzza, Stephanie Van Dam, Karen Stanley, Madonna Lazo-Smith, Lexy Land, Roberta Zwier, Libby Smith, Janna Mukherjee, Mary Hopper, Ayesha Santos (the wonderful illustrator for this book too!). Your friendship means the absolute world to me!

Thank you to my family; Cody, Olivia, Harrison, Dean, June, my parents Nirwan and Renno, Lia, Feby, Tom, Sandra, for always being there for me, whether its to help out, watch kids, make meals, send funny messages or try to remind me of time zones and TV shows. I love you. Thank you!

Writing this book was a profoundly surprising experience. After the success of my first book, *Nourish Your Body: A 30-Day Healthy and Delicious Meal Plan*, I knew that I wanted to write another book. However, while I had a multitude of ideas for books, my heart just wasn't in any of them.

Until, I got shingles.

Once I recovered from shingles and had a moment to process what happened, I realized that my healing journey was what I needed to write about. Once that decision was made, everything seemed to fall into place. I was able to write easily and freely. I was able to create recipes that people loved and kept asking if the recipes were going to be in the next book. It seemed as if everything just happened at the right time.

Here's what I learned: everything that happens can serve a greater purpose, if we choose to see it that way.

What will you choose today?

Renata

References

1. TED Talks. (11 June 2011). How to stop screwing yourself over | Mel Robbins | TEDxSF (Video), https://youtu.be/Lp7E973zozc

2. Klinghardt Institute, Klinghardt Institute – *The Heart of Healing*, accessed 16 June 2022, https://klinghardtinstitute.com/

3. National Library of Medicine, National Center for Biotechnology Information, *The Impact of Nutrition and Environmental Epigenetics on Human Health and Disease*, accessed 6 April 2022, https://www.ncbi.nlm.nih.gov/pmc/articles/PMC6275017/

4. UCLA Health, *If You Want to Boost Immunity, Look to the Gut*, accessed 16 June 2022, https://connect.uclahealth.org/2021/03/19/want-to-boost-immunity-look-to-the-gut/#:~:text=70%25%20of%20the%20immune%20system,diet%20affects%20the%20immune%20system

5. National Library of Medicine, National Center for Biotechnology Information, *Alterations of the Gut Microbiome and Metabolome in Alcoholic Liver Disease*, accessed 16 June 2022, https://www.ncbi.nlm.nih.gov/pmc/articles/PMC4231516/

6. National Library of Medicine, National Center for Biotechnology Information, *Whole-grain intake is favorably associated with metabolic risk factors for type 2 diabetes and cardiovascular disease in the Framingham Offspring Study*, accessed 6 April 2022, http://www.ncbi.nlm.nih.gov/pubmed/12145012

7. National Library of Medicine, National Center for Biotechnology Information, *Understanding nutrition, depression and mental illness,* accessed 17 June 2022, https://www.ncbi.nlm.nih.gov/pmc/articles/PMC2738337/

8. Public Library of Science One, *The Weight of a Guilty Conscience: Subjective Body Weight as an Embodiment of Guilt,* accessed 27 April 2022, https://journals.plos.org/plosone/article/file?id=10.1371/journal.pone.0069546&type=printable

9. National Library of Medicine, National Center for Biotechnology Information, *The Impact of Stress on Body Function: A Review,* accessed 13 April 2022, https://www.ncbi.nlm.nih.gov/pmc/articles/PMC5579396/

10. Health Plus, *10 Conditions Linked to Stress,* accessed 27 April 2022, https://www.mountelizabeth.com.sg/healthplus/article/health-conditions-linked-to-stress

11. National Library of Medicine, National Center for Biotechnology Information, *Stress, depression, diet, and the gut microbiota: human-bacteria interactions at the core of psychoneuroimmunology and nutrition,* accessed 13 April 2022, https://www.ncbi.nlm.nih.gov/pmc/articles/PMC7213601/

12. National Library of Medicine, National Center for Biotechnology Information, *Gut Microbiome and Depression: How Microbes Affect the Way We Think,* accessed 13 July 2022, https://www.ncbi.nlm.nih.gov/pmc/articles/PMC7510518/

13. National Library of Medicine, National Center for Biotechnology Information, *Neuropharmacology of N,N-Dimethyltryptamine,* accessed 20 April 2022, https://www.ncbi.nlm.nih.gov/pmc/articles/PMC5048497/

14. National Library of Medicine, National Center for Biotechnology Information, *Effect of uninostril yoga breathing on brain hemodynamics: A functional near-infrared spectroscopy study,* accessed 20 April 2022, https://www.ncbi.nlm.nih.gov/pmc/articles/PMC4728953/

15. National Library of Medicine, National Center for Biotechnology Information, *Energy Medicine: Current Status and Future Perspectives,* accessed 8 June 2022, https://www.ncbi.nlm.nih.gov/pmc/articles/PMC6396053/

16. National Library of Medicine, National Center for Biotechnology Information, *Evaluation of the antifungal efficacy of different concentrations of Curcuma longa on Candida albicans: An invitro study,* accessed 20 July 2022, https://www.ncbi.nlm.nih.gov/pmc/articles/PMC6714268/#:~:text=From%20the%20results%20of%20our,fungicidal%20effects%20at%20higher%20concentrations

Visit
http://www.
nourishwithrenata.com/
healyourbodymind
andspirit
for exclusive bonuses
and videos.

www.ingramcontent.com/pod-product-compliance
Lightning Source LLC
Chambersburg PA
CBHW052113030426
42335CB00025B/2957